Completely fascinating reading. I literally could not put this book down.

This incredibly important and exciting information is presented in an easy to read and under-stand format, which flows well and does not disappoint on any level. This is what the world of medicine should look like.

This book should be offered in every first year of medical school so that prospective doctors have the opportunity to learn how true healing takes place, rather than simply being trained to suppress symptoms without addressing the underlying causes of illness, imbalances and dis-eases in our bodies. It should be required reading for every traditional allopathic physician and every patient on the planet.

If you are interested in your health, you must read this book. It opens you up to a new world, literally. But buyer beware… this book may alter your beliefs about the established medical system in this country, bringing you into true illumination and precipitate a paradigm shift of unparalleled magnitude.

The only problem I had with it…. It left me wanting more!

The value of the information in this book and the understanding to be gained by reading it, far exceeds its cost. Buy one for everyone you know!

—**HOLLY J. PERRY,** Human Energy Field Therapist

At last! For those seeking an alternative medicine doctor, this book has it all. Dr. Edward C. Kondrot, MD and ophthalmologist, has brought together doctors from all disciplines and inter-viewed them on their areas of interest.

This is a book that not only allows the person to become educated in what kinds of alternative medicine are out there, but what these disciplines or therapies are, what they do to help a person who is sick. And with education, the person can make a solid decision as to what appeals to them from the "tools" that are out there but little known about.

—**LINDSAY MCKENNA,** *New York Times* best-selling author

Such a wealth of information! This book should be available in every library, medical office, and hospital as a reference for the many patients who are diagnosed with or suffer from painful and debilitating conditions. I thought I knew the world of alternative medicine, but I learned so much more in this book. All the techniques and methods are compelling to read, but, in the end, the most important message is that no matter what your prognosis or how intense your pain, there is something that can be done to help you. Knowing this is healing in itself, and now we know how to find this help. Thank you, Dr. Kondrot, for shining the light on these wonderful healers.

—**GLORIA ST JOHN, MA, MBA,** Classical Homeopath, Medical Researcher and Writer

This book offers hope for those who have been told that there is no hope. It provides the reader with an understanding of the concepts of homeopathy through the experiences and knowledge of the leading alternative doctors involved in this important work in a reader-friendly format.

—**CHRISTINE KONDROT,** Public Relations Consultant

Dr. Kondrot's interviews with these real healers is an eye and mind opening experience. Since retiring 13 years ago, I began my search for better ways to maintain my health. I found the website of the Arizona Homeopathic and Integrative Medical Association (AHIMA). In turn, I have found physicians such as Dr. Charles Schwengel in Mesa, AZ, and Dr. Kondrot in Phoenix, all members of AHIMA. These doctors have helped to treat and teach me how to maintain my health in these later years. Reading the accomplishments and treatments that these caring physicians have developed, improved upon, and use in their respective practices gives me great confidence in what they can do for me and all of their patients. I am putting into practice the ozone and oxygenation protocols previously described to me by Dr. Kondrot and now in this book. Thanks to all of you!

Our governments have failed to maintain our wonderful country's environment and still stifle rather than encourage efforts to accept and promote the wonderful healing work of these 20 dedicated healers as well as the hundreds or thousands of other doctors, dentists and other therapists who heal rather than succumb to greed. I am certain my body is thankful for not receiving any pharmaceuticals as treatment for "disease" anymore.

—**LOUIS DRUMMOND**

Learn How the TOP 20 ALTERNATIVE DOCTORS in AMERICA Can Improve Your HEALTH

Abram Ber, MD(H) · Dennis Courtney, MD · Gabriel Cousens, MD, MD(H) ·
Lee Cowden, MD, MD(H) · Garry Gordon, DO, MD, MD(H) · Edward C. Kondrot, MD, MD(H) ·
James Lemire, MD · Ruth Tan Lim, MD, MD(H) · Michael Margolis, DDS · Dorothy Merritt, MD
· Nicholas J. Meyer, DDS · David Nebbeling, DO · Karl Robinson, MD · Robert Rowen, MD ·
Charles Schwengel, DO, DO(H) · Frank Shallenberger, MD, HMD · Bruce Shelton, MD, MD(H)
· Mark Starr, MD, MD(H) · David Steenblock, DO · Jerald Tennant, MD, MD(H)

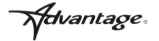

Published by Advantage, Charleston, South Carolina.
Member of Advantage Media Group.

ADVANTAGE is a registered trademark and the Advantage colophon is a trademark of Advantage Media Group, Inc.

Printed in the United States of America.

ISBN: 978-1-59932-476-0
LCCN: 2014932736

This publication is designed to provide accurate and authoritative information in regard to the subject matter covered. It is sold with the understanding that the publisher is not engaged in rendering legal, accounting, or other professional services. If legal advice or other expert assistance is required, the services of a competent professional person should be sought.

Advantage Media Group is proud to be a part of the Tree Neutral® program. Tree Neutral offsets the number of trees consumed in the production and printing of this book by taking proactive steps such as planting trees in direct proportion to the number of trees used to print books. To learn more about Tree Neutral, please visit www.treeneutral.com. To learn more about Advantage's commitment to being a responsible steward of the environment, please visit www.advantagefamily.com/green

Advantage Media Group is a publisher of business, self-improvement, and professional development books and online learning. We help entrepreneurs, business leaders, and professionals share their Stories, Passion, and Knowledge to help others Learn & Grow. Do you have a manuscript or book idea that you would like us to consider for publishing? Please visit advantagefamily.com or call 1.866.775.1696.

This book is dedicated to my wonderful wife Ly.

Acknowledgements

I want to thank the Top 20 Alternative Doctors who have contributed to this book.

Fourteen of them are medical doctors; four are osteopathic doctors; and two are dentists. They are located around the country, with a concentration in Arizona and Texas. Most have a national, if not international, practice and serve patients both locally and from afar. The stories of how and why they embraced alternative and holistic therapies, after undergoing training in conventional medicine or dentistry, are almost as compelling as their discussion of techniques and modalities. On behalf of patients everywhere, I am especially grateful to these creative and selfless practitioners for affirming that, "There is always hope — regardless of your pain or your diagnosis." Unfortunately we often need to look beyond the limits of conventional medicine to hear this message. Fortunately, we now know where to look.

Readers will appreciate the list of books written by the doctors featured in this book. It appears at the end of the book and will be a rich resource for those who want to learn more about the alternative therapies as practiced by the contributing doctors.

I would like to thank all the members on the Board of the Arizona Homeopathic and Integrative Medical Association and the executive secretary Lisa Platt.

I extend thanks to Gloria St. John for her major contribution in editing this book. As a practicing homeopath and medical researcher and editor, she brings a mix of talents that made the chapters in this book consistent and easy to understand for every type of reader. My cousin Christine Kondrot provided the final copy editing; I can always trust her sharp eye to produce an impeccable manuscript that reflects the intent of the authors.

The staff of KFNX Talk Radio gave me the opportunity to broadcast and give voice to the doctors in this book. Those interviews formed the basis of this material.

Special thanks to Advantage Media Group for accomplishing the task of putting the printed material into book form.

Lastly, my greatest appreciation goes to my wonderful wife, Ly, who supported me in this important project.

Edward C. Kondrot, MD, MD(H), CCH, DHt

Contents

Preface

When I became President of the Arizona Homeopathic and Integrative Medical Association (AHIMA), I was honored to represent a much-esteemed group of alternative doctors. These individuals work tirelessly to bring you the latest in treatments that will restore your health. Most of these treatments are approaches that are not included in conventional medicine.

My first reaction as President of AHIMA was to ask how the wonderful, unselfish, and creative work of these members might come into greater awareness. These doctors are not always known to the many patients who are seeking safe and effective alternative treatments to restore their health. I wanted to bridge the gap and allow more patients to meet these incredible healers.

I decided that the best way to accomplish this was to interview each doctor to learn how they made the transition to alternative therapies, what makes their practice unique, what types of conditions they treat, and patients they serve. I changed my radio show, *Healthy Vision Talk Radio*, to the *Top Alternative Doctors of America*, and, over a period of months, interviewed each one of these special individuals who are making a marked difference in health care in America. Then, I realized that more people could learn about them if I compiled a book of these interviews. You have it in your hands.

You may wonder why you have not heard of some of these doctors. Well, these clinicians are quietly working in the trenches, helping thousands of people without the national recognition of pop TV doctors or publicity. Several began their journey when their own health deteriorated and did not respond to conventional therapies. This happened to me also, and this experience makes us empathize with people who have tried everything to regain their heath but are still sick.

How would you go about finding a doctor who can help you the most? Reading this book is almost like a consultation with these specialists in alternative and innovative therapies. One of them has observed that we are all prone to disease. Some of you may be ill right now, or you may have a loved one or friend who has been given a hopeless sentence from conventional medicine. Or you may be healthy now but want to keep resources handy, just in case. Open the pages of this book and receive valuable information to improve and keep your health. Remember, hope is a component of the healing journey.

To your good health!

DR. EDWARD KONDROT, MD, MD(H), CCH, DHT
President of the Arizona Homeopathic and Integrative Medical Association
Clinic Director of the American Medical College of Homeopathy
Host of *Healthy Vision Talk Radio*
Director of the Healing the Eye and Wellness Center
www.HealingTheEye.com

Foreword

By Todd Rowe, MD, MD(H), CCH, DHT

Explore the Secrets of Health and Disease through Learning from America's Top Alternative Medicine Doctors

In this book, each of these physicians describes their journey from being a conventional doctor to becoming one of the leading alternative medicine doctors in the country. Many describe key moments in their lives where their thinking and awareness of both health and disease became transformed.

Learn from Dr. Abram Ber how to reduce the risks of acquiring parasites and preventing the spread of Lyme disease. Explore with Dr. Gabriel Cousens the secrets to reducing the effects of diabetes. Discover ways to improve your eyesight and prevent blindness with Dr. Edward Kondrot. Discern methods to reduce your cardiac risk and to better choose heart medications with Dr. Dorothy Merritt. Listen to Dr. Nicholas Meyer as he reveals the dangers of root canals and mercury fillings and shares the health consequences of misaligned bite. Catch the fire of Dr. Karl Robinson's passion for classical homeopathy and learn how it can transform lives. Listen to a master alternative practitioner, Dr. Bruce Shelton, as he shares the secret to removing mold toxicity and reveals the health consequences of scars. Study with Dr. Robert Rowen as he shares methods to detox from mercury and do chelation therapies for heavy metals from home. Learn from Dr. James Lemire as he discusses methods to reduce conventional medications, holistically treat cardiac disease, and effectively use bioidentical hormones.

Dr. Charlie Schwengel, an osteopathic doctor, focuses on providing alternative choices in the treatment of cancer, through getting to root causes and using herbal medicine and homeopathy. Dr. Garry Gordon describes how his F.I.G.H.T. for Your Health program offers a simple and safe way to deal with illness and disease for optimum health and anti-aging. Dr. Dennis Courtney shares his "treatment tripod" which includes treatment of deficiencies, toxicities, and diminishing profusion for best results. Dr. Lee Cowden, president of the Academy of Comprehensive Medicine, explores his secrets of success in the treatment of Lyme disease, using a variety of techniques. Dr. Ruth Lim, a pediatric specialist, emphasizes the importance of nutrition for infants, importance of gut health, and plant-based diets for adults.

Dr. Mike Margolis, a biological dentist describes the hidden health problems associated with root canals, how mercury fillings cause toxicity, and simple tests you can do to determine if you are at risk for mercury toxicity from your fillings. Dr. David Nebbling, an osteopathic doctor, uses cranial manipulation, prolotherapy, oxidative treatments, and nutrition in his holistic approaches to the treatment of cancer. Dr. Frank Shallenberger, a lifetime achievement award winner with the Arizona Homeopathic and Integrative Medicine Association, explores oxidative therapies and their cure of many chronic diseases.

Dr. Mark Starr, author of several books on thyroid disorders, describes the hidden epidemic of thyroid deficiency in both adults and children, and how this is commonly missed in conventional medicine. Dr. David Steenblock, author of several books on stem cell therapy, describes a secret to increasing stem cell levels in your body and the amazing results that stem cell therapies can produce in the regeneration of damaged tissues. Dr. Jerry Tennant, author of *Healing is Voltage*, shares his journey to health and how it led to the creation of the Tenant Biomodulator that can restore healthy voltages to tissues with electron deficiency in the body.

Who are the Experts in Alternative Medicine?

Because alternative medicine involves a diversity of disciplines and styles of training, it has been difficult for the public to determine the quality of practitioners. This is particularly true for medical and osteopathic doctors. This book provides a listing of some of the top alternative medicine doctors in the United States. It describes their work and their approaches to promoting health and preventing disease. The assembly of these experts and their work into a single volume has been a major effort and is of great potential benefit to the public.

It has been both my privilege and honor to have worked as a colleague with these doctors and to observe their incredible results firsthand. Over the 25 years that I have been in practice, I have had many opportunities to work with them as colleagues, in seminars, and as faculty members at our college. I have been able to observe firsthand the incredible successes that they experience daily in their practices.

The material in this book has been generated from a series of interviews that were conducted during 2013 by Dr. Edward Kondrot. Dr. Kondrot is now the president of the Arizona Homeopathic and Integrative Medicine Association, faculty member at the American Medical College of Homeopathy, and the clinic director for the Integrative Medicine Clinic at the American Medical College of Homeopathy. Many of these doctors work at the AMCH Integrative Medicine Clinic, offering reduced fee services to the public. As clinic director, Dr. Kondrot has had a unique opportunity to work with each of these doctors and to know firsthand the high quality of their work. The essential discoveries that they have made come shining through these interviews.

What is Alternative Medicine?

This book refers repeatedly to both alternative and integrative medicine. What is alternative and integrative medicine?

Alternative medicine can be defined as any of a broad range of healing approaches not used in conventional Western medicine. Many are holistic and many also emphasize prevention and education. Alternative therapies include amongst others:

Acupuncture/Chinese Medicine/Qigong	Hydrotherapy
Aromatherapy	Jin Shin Jujitsu
Ayurvedic Medicine	Massage
Chelation	Meditation
Chiropractry	Mind/Body Medicine
Colon Therapy	Naturopathy
Energy Medicine	Orthomolecular Medicine
Environmental Medicine	Osteopathy
Flower Essences	Reiki
Herbal Medicine	Rolphing
Holistic Dentistry	Spiritual Healing
Homeopathy	Therapeutic Touch
	Yoga

Though considered alternative in the West, such medicine is the main source of health care for up to 80% of people in less-developed countries. Alternative medicine approaches may offer treatments in areas where conventional approaches have not succeeded.

What is integrative medicine? The concept of integrative medicine is very popular in the country today and has become somewhat of a common term. In this process, it has taken on many meanings depending on the group defining it. Integrative medicine is a new health care discipline being established by United States medical schools seeking to combine ideas and practices of Western medicine and alternative medicine. Perhaps the best definition that I have come across is the following:

> Integrative Medicine is the practice of medicine that reaffirms the importance of relationship between practitioner and patient, focuses on the whole person, is informed by evidence, and makes use of all appropriate therapeutic approaches, providers, and disciplines to achieve optimal health and healing (ACCAHC).

The Arizona Homeopathic and Integrative Medicine Association

All of the doctors in this book are affiliated with the Arizona Homeopathic and Integrative Medicine Association (www.arizonahomeopathic.org), and many are licensed through the Arizona State Board of Homeopathic and Integrative Medicine Examiners (www.azhomeopathbd.az.gov). This board includes within its scope the practice of acupuncture, chelation, homeopathy, minor surgery, neuromuscular integration, nutrition, orthomolecular therapy, and pharmaceutical medicine.

American Medical College of Homeopathy

Many of the doctors in this book are on faculty at the American Medical College of Homeopathy (www.AMCofH.org). This college is a community partner with the Arizona Homeopathic and Integrative Medicine Association. AMCH is a non-profit college that has existed for 15 years in Phoenix, Arizona. The college is a center of excellence in homeopathic education, clinical care, and research. It also provides education in integrative medicine, offers an integrative medicine clinic, and promotes quality research in integrative medicine.

AMCH Programs

AMCH offers a variety of programs that provide education in alternative medicine (www.AMCofH.org).

HOMEOPATHIC PRACTITIONER PROGRAM: 1,200 hour, three-year, part-time program; campus and on-line options; weekend based. Maryann Ivons, ND, is the program director.

VITHOULKAS COMPREHENSIVE PROGRAM IN CLASSICAL HOMEOPATHY: 600 hour, two-year, part-time program; weekday evening based; campus and online options. Dan Horvath, CCH, is the program director.

ACUTE CARE PROGRAM: 40 hour, six-month, part-time program; campus, distance learning, and online options. Debbie Noah, CCH, is the program director.

INTEGRATIVE MEDICINE PROGRAM: 35 hour, six-month, part-time program; online option only. Bruce Shelton, MD, MD(H), is the program director.

PRECEPTORSHIP PROGRAMS: These range from one day to one month and are targeted at medical doctors, osteopathic doctors, nurse practitioners, and chiropractors interested in studying homeopathic medicine. Carole Eastman is the program director.

AMCH Medical Center

AMCH offers a variety of teaching and research clinics that are open to the public at reduced fee prices (http://www.amcofh.org/medical-center/clinical-services).

INTEGRATIVE MEDICINE CLINIC: This clinic offers reduced fee integrative medicine services for the public. Edward Kondrot, MD, MD(H) is the clinic director. This clinic offers reduced fee services to the community.

CHRONIC CARE HOMEOPATHIC CLINIC: This clinic provides reduced fee services for patients with chronic health care problems. Mary Grace Warner, MD, MD(H) is the clinic director.

ACUTE CARE HOMEOPATHIC CLINIC: This clinic provides reduced fee walk-in services for patients with acute health problems. Maryann Ivons, ND, is the clinic director.

HIV/AIDS FREE CLINIC: This clinic offers free services for HIV/AIDS patients at the Southwest HIV/AIDS Center. The clinic director is Mario Fontes, LAc, CCH.

WOMEN'S HEALTH CLINIC: This clinic offers free services for women at the Fresh Start Women's Health Center. The clinic director is Debbie Noah, CCH.

AMCH Department of Research

The American Medical College of Homeopathy provides a Center of Excellence for homeopathic research in North America. This includes homeopathic research education, homeopathic proving trials, homeopathic community research, homeopathic community trial research, and homeopathic basic science research.

Proving Research

AMCH has conducted 23 Homeopathic Proving Trials since 1993. All have been published in monograph form and submitted/included in the major homeopathic software. A listing of provings conducted can be found at www.amcofh.org/research/proving-trials. AMCH provings are consistent with HPUS and NANHE (North American Network of Homeopathic Education) national proving standards.

Community Research

AMCH has conducted a series of comprehensive North America surveys on homeopathic practice. These have included homeopathic practitioner surveys (2006, 2013), homeopathic patient surveys (2007, 2014) and homeopathic education surveys. The results of these surveys can be found at www.amcofh.org/research/community.

Clinical Trial Research

The AMCH Research Director has conducted multiple clinical trials. AMCH has participated in Clinical Trial Research and is available to conduct a range of Clinical Trials including Open Label Trials.

Basic Science Research

AMCH has helped to conduct basic science research exploring the mechanism of action of homeopathic medicines.

Introduction to Homeopathic Research Program

AMCH offers a 20-hour online asynchronous program in homeopathic research entitled *Introduction to Homeopathic Research*. Dr. Iris Bell is the director for the program. Faculty includes Dr. Bell, Dr. Todd Rowe, Dr. Mary Koithan, and Dr. Bonnie Phelps. Continuing Education (CME) credits are available.

Abram Ber, MD, MD(H)

SCOTTSDALE, ARIZONA

Interviewed August 11, 2013

1. People who eat out frequently have a greater chance of acquiring parasites.

2. The inside of our homes has to become a total green zone.

3. Lyme disease can be spread from one person to another.

DR. KONDROT: Dr. Abram Ber is one of the co-founders of the Arizona Homeopathic Association and is considered to be the father of our great organization. Share a little bit about your medical career and how you became one of the top alternative doctors.

DR. BER: First of all, I graduated from medical school at McGill University in Montreal, Canada, where I lived a good part of my life. Subsequent to that, I interned, did a year of residency in internal medicine and three years of residency in anesthesiology, and became a board-certified anesthesiologist. I practiced only anesthesiology for a couple of years. Then, I took over the general medicine practice of a physician who was deceased. While I was in the general practice, using allopathic modalities, I had never heard of the words holistic or alternative.

Somewhere in 1975, which is apparently an important year for quite a few holistic practitioners, a patient gave me a book on vitamin E, which was written by the Schute brothers from Ontario. They were experts on vitamin E. Right after

I read the book, a young woman with a leg swollen from phlebitis came into my office. I said, "I've just read a book on vitamin E. I've never used it before, but I'll give you a prescription for it."

She agreed and went to the pharmacy to buy the vitamin E. When she returned some weeks later, her leg was almost normal. I was astounded. I knew about vitamin E as a vitamin, of course, but nothing else about it had been taught in medical school.

That was the awakening. Subsequently, I asked my wife to go to the health food store to get me some information on garlic. When the man who owned the store learned that I was a medical doctor, he gave her a book for me to read. He asked that I return it when I was finished, and he would lend me another. This man gave me an entire education. That was the beginning: a patient and a health food storeowner.

DR. KONDROT: It's interesting that most of us in alternative medicine really don't learn our art from medical school. Interestingly, we learn more from our patients.

DR. BER: I went to the hospital where I was working and asked about the use of vitamins. No one knew what I was talking about. I started to incorporate vitamins, minerals, and other modalities while I was still practicing in Montreal. In 1977, I relocated from Montreal to Phoenix to work at the Association for Research and Enlightenment (ARE) Clinic in Phoenix.

This was a clinic that was run by Drs. Bill and Gladys McGary who are both holistic medical doctors with many years of experience. They had this very well known, fabulous clinic, which was associated with Edgar Cayce, who was the greatest medical intuitive in the United States.

Subsequent to that, I opened my own office in Phoenix. Next, I attended a conference in San Francisco, given by a Dr. Voll. That was the most significant conference I ever attended because, as a result of that conference, it struck me that what he was doing was unique. He had been using a device called a Dermatron, which was an electrodermal device. With this device, he was able to access information from the body accurately using no X-rays or blood tests. Because he was a medical doctor, he was able to prove the accuracy of his work. Soon after, I bought a Dermatron, and I still use the one that I bought 34 years ago. I have become adept at using it because I do all the testing myself.

DR. KONDROT: Before we go into any more detail about the Dermatron, talk a little bit about your experience at the ARE Clinic. What did you learn during that time period that has influenced your approach to treating disease and evaluating patients?

DR. BER: That was a very important part of the paradigm shift in my thinking. Of course, the ARE Clinic used regular medical modalities like any other medical doctor would, but they incorporated information from the Edgar Cayce readings, which he did while in a state of trance. People would come to him with medical problems, for which there weren't adequate answers in the years that he was giving readings in the '20s and '30s, not that we have so many adequate answers today. He was able to go into a trance, and in that state he would give the precise etiology and physiology of a person's condition. He also gave a deeper reason for people's illnesses. He'd be able to tell the person what the problem was and where to find the medicine that would relieve the condition. He was accurate, and he helped countless people. People came from all over the world to get a reading from Edgar Cayce. The work of Edgar Cayce still continues at the ARE Foundation, which is in Virginia Beach, Virginia, and publishes a phenomenal, holistic magazine called *Venture Inward*.

DR. KONDROT: I also have an interest in the work of Edgar Cayce. I have recordings of all of his readings. Often, I do a search of eye diseases and review some of the readings that Edgar Cayce did, and I often get ideas to help my patients.

I wonder if you could explain more about the Dermatron.

DR. BER: A good part of my practice is based on the use of the Dermatron in assessing a patient's condition. The Dermatron is an electrodermal device.

Dr. Voll found that over acupuncture points there is significantly less skin resistance than over skin in general. As you introduce something within the circuitry of the Dermatron, if that substance is a problem for the patient, then there is an indicator that shows as a change in the electrical resistance. It's not unlike muscle testing and kinesiology. The difference is that when I do my testing, I do it without knowing what I test. In other words, the label is on the bottom of the vials I use so that I cannot influence the results with my mind. It's easy to influence. It took me years to adapt to this technique and hide the answer from my direct knowledge. One problem with doing muscle testing is that, if you know what you're testing and have a predisposition to a certain result, you may get the wrong answer. I'm interested in getting the right answer.

DR. KONDROT: Do you have a certain systematic approach? Do you begin by testing certain things?

DR. BER: It depends on the patient's problem. If a patient comes to me for an acute infection, I want to know if it's a virus, bacteria, or fungus. I test quickly to be able to focus on the exact infection that I need to address.

First of all, I take a history so that I know where to focus. Over the years, I have acquired pathological organisms. They are not homeopathic. They're actually bacteriological extracts that I obtained over years of collecting parasites, viruses, bacteria, and fungi, and then making serial dilutions of them. The work that I do is based very much on what Dr. Bill Ray does, which is the serial dilution neutralization technique. That means that the extract of, let's say, Epstein-Barr virus is diluted.

The first dilution is made by adding 8cc of water to 2cc of the concentrated extract, e.g. dust. The second dilution is made by adding 8cc of water to the first dilution, and so on. It's a serial dilution. What I do is find the exact neutralizing solution, which the patient takes under the tongue. It's a method that's very precise and very accurate. It works.

To give you an example, recently a woman consulted me with symptoms of severe digestive problems. I diagnosed her with a parasite and told her that this parasite was *Ascaris lumbricoides*, which is roundworm. I treated her and then told her it was probably from her dog. The vet tested the dog and found roundworms.

Over the years, some people I tested and told that they had Epstein-Barr virus or Valley Fever had a blood test, and it showed that they had those conditions. My approach has been proven quite accurate.

As the years progressed, the problems that patients have, have become more and more complicated compared to when I first came to Phoenix in the '70s to work at the clinic. It's like we're living on another planet. It's not the same. We now have organisms that didn't exist when I went to medical school. There was no

Lyme disease when I went to McGill in the '60s. There was no *Mycoplasma*. We don't know where these organisms come from or how they have been introduced to the population.

The general medical profession doesn't recognize the severity of the infections that come with Lyme disease and mycoplasma. They pay little attention because the blood tests that they do don't pick it up. They tell people that they don't have Lyme disease.

These patients go to the so-called Lyme literate doctors who are persecuted all over America for doing the work that needs to be done accurately. They're doing it effectively to help patients. Their licenses are being taken away because they're treating Lyme disease, which the medical profession says is not common. When I do a Dermatron test on patients with chronic disease, the majority have a major organism that belongs to the Lyme disease family. These infections are not only from the original *Borrelia*, but also the infections of *Ehrlichia, Babesia, Bartonella,* and *Mycoplasma*. All of these exist and are creating disease in many people.

DR. KONDROT: What do you think is the reason for this change in pathology? You mentioned that these things didn't exist when you went to medical school. Do you have any ideas or thoughts on their origin?

DR. BER: I've read the stories about biological experiments out in the East. I don't know. It could be Earth changes, the global warming effect, the use of pesticides all over this country, or genetically modified foods that were developed in 1996 and that didn't exist before.

There's the new technology of electromagnetics that surround us, like cell phone towers. It's not just your little cell phone you're holding in your hand, it's the cell phone towers that are hiding all over the place that are wiping us out. It's now a major calamity. All of these together are allowing the growth of organisms that didn't exist before. People wonder why we have 1.5 million children who are autistic in this country. Some of the answers could be the vaccinations and the general deterioration of the environment.

Not one of us escapes this lifetime without problems. Infections are universal. Even if a person is healthy, there's some infection in the body. When I see a new patient, the first thing I do is test to determine the predominant infectious agent. Is it bacteria, virus, fungus, or parasite? I deal with that first.

I've also been very influenced by the work and research of Dr. Dietrich Klinghardt who is internationally recognized for his treatment of chronic pain and illness. Let's say I find parasites as a predominant problem in a patient. Parasites are very common. In the general medical population, they are hardly ever diagnosed. If a patient has severe and chronic gastroenteritis, their doctor will do a culture of the stool and check for bacteria. This is pretty accurate. The results will come back as salmonella, E. coli, or staph. What about the parasites? Occasionally they will do a blood test for giardia. It pretty much stops there.

A world-class parasitologist, Dr. Omar Amin, is here in Arizona, but that is a rarity. Besides him, there's nobody. The people who are trained in lab work are not trained to be able to diagnose parasites. I am able to get information about parasites using the Dermatron. I test for the common parasites that one sees in this country. Blastocystis is one. It's innocuous enough, but it can cause problems. We have a natural therapy for parasites, which I then administer. Occasionally, I also use some medication for a short period of time. We use both medication and herbal remedies to get rid of the parasites.

1. People who eat out frequently have a greater chance of acquiring parasites.

I'm emphasizing this so people realize that parasites are very common, because we are now a global community. People who work in restaurants are often from other countries, and they have brought the parasites from their homeland. Their hygiene may not be the best, but, even if their hygiene is very good, my finding is that people who eat out frequently have a greater chance of acquiring parasites.

DR. KONDROT: Dr. Ber, don't you also think that our immune system is becoming weaker and allowing parasites to grow more readily in our bodies?

DR. BER: There's no question that the immune system is getting weaker. It's getting weaker because we have too much to handle. We are not adapted to handle so many chemicals or air pollution. There was no air pollution 100 years ago. Air pollution has been demonstrated to cause hardening of the arteries. This is an amazing thing. Of course, we realize that it causes lung problems, but it also causes coronary disease and many other problems.

2. The inside of our homes has to become a total green zone.

This is what we have to do inside our homes. The inside of our homes has to become a total green zone. You cannot use any chemicals at all in the house. You can clean only with water and vinegar. If you need additional things, you can buy something at a health food store. Do not use toxic chemicals, which are then emitted into the air. Some people have a monthly service to spray pesticides in the house to prevent cockroaches and the other things. This is why we have an epidemic of diseases in our immune system. The immune system is really under duress. What we have to do is to diminish the total load upon us. We cannot do anything about the outside air or the workplace, but we can do everything about our house. Absolutely nothing must come in your house.

Eat organic food. Some foods are more contaminated than others; apples and strawberries are really bad news. There are certain vegetables that don't have to be organic such as asparagus and avocados. If you're going to eat chicken, get organic chicken. Commercially raised chickens, as well as livestock, are fed genetically modified corn or soy.

Wheat, which is not genetically modified, has been tampered with. The wheat has been hybridized and changed into something else. That's why so many people are gluten sensitive. Gluten sensitivity wasn't that common 25 or 30 years ago.

Occasionally there are people who have Celiac disease and truly are gluten sensitive, but now it's very common for patients to tell me that they cannot eat bread. This is what has happened because our immune systems are being systematically depleted. We're under attack, and it's getting difficult to stay healthy.

It's difficult to keep our children healthy because, if you take a child to a pediatrician, they get one immunization after another. We are not adapted for mass immunization. Never in the history of mankind has this existed. It's very likely that many children have become very sick.

I don't know the whole story about autism and whether it's due only to vaccinations. It may not be. It may be also environmental pollution, heavy metals in the air such as mercury, and other things that are causing the complication with autism. But, one thing is certain; they give too many vaccinations at one time. They're giving vaccinations for diseases that don't exist anymore.

If you cut your foot and go to the emergency room, they will give you a tetanus injection. Why? They give it to prevent tetanus, but the fact is that in the whole of the United States, there are only a few cases of tetanus per year. The tetanus vaccination can make you sick for the rest of your life. It affects the brain and the nervous system. This is what we have with traditional medicine.

When a patient comes to me, I try to diminish the load on their immune system. Of course, I will treat food allergies, but I'll address the main infection first. Then when they come back for another visit, I'll check again to see if they have a bacterium. Very often, they have one called the Lyme organism. Lyme disease, which didn't exist when I went to medical school, is now so prevalent that it affects all ages.

3. Lyme disease can be spread from one person to another.

I have had children come in with allergies. They don't have the specific symptoms that make you think about Lyme disease. Of course, Lyme disease can cause neurological problems like muscular dystrophy (MS) and even heart disease and myocarditis. Children come in, and when I test them with a Dermatron for infections, they will frequently show up with Lyme disease. It's a puzzler. How did they get it? It looks like Lyme disease can be spread from the pregnant mother across the placenta into the newborn. Lyme disease

originally had to do with getting a bite from a tick from a deer. People say, "I haven't ever been bitten by a tick." It turns out that mosquitoes and fleas can also be full of Lyme organisms. In addition to that, it can be spread from one person to another. Enough people now have it that it's spreading from one person to another.

If I find it early, and the person is not yet sick with it, I can treat it using homeopathic remedies that address specific Lyme organisms and transfer factors that are made from cow colostrum by injecting them and giving them the organism. We use transfer factors and homeopathy, and the results are extremely effective and very gratifying. I don't use antibiotics in the treatment of Lyme, although many holistic doctors treat Lyme using antibiotics, even intravenous antibiotics.

I am very grateful to the Creator who put me in touch with therapies that don't require invasion and antibiotics that upset the bowel flora and create new diseases. Patients get better. Two months ago, I saw a patient referred to me by a local physician. She had acute arthritis so severe that she could barely walk. She was at the end of the road. I tested her using the Dermatron and found that she had mycoplasma. I gave her the treatment for mycoplasma. Week by week, she started to get better. I just saw her two days ago in my office, and she is dramatically improved. Before, she was incapacitated to the point of not knowing how to pursue life. I addressed the mycoplasma using natural therapies.

A very common problem that shows up in my testing is mold and fungi. They're so prominent; it's unbelievable. Dr. Ritchie Shoemaker is the number-one authority in this country on mold. He has written about it, and he's right on. People have all kinds of problems as a result of mold. They're not always aware where the mold came from. They're not aware that there is or was a water leak in the house, although frequently that is the start of the problem.

I just want to mention the two foods people should not eat because they are almost universally moldy. One is peanuts. Every kid in this country loves peanut butter, but it is afflicted with aspergillus mold, which is a known cause of aflatoxin contamination. The other food that has so many problems is corn. Corn is genetically modified. That's one problem, but corn also has a mold problem. If patients have a mold problem, I ask them if they eat these foods. If they do, I tell them to desist. That's enough. They have options other than peanut butter. We have almond butter and other kinds of nut butters.

What I do is I find the exact mold that a person has and give them a dilution that neutralizes their mold sensitivity.

The most common mold or fungus in Arizona is associated with Valley Fever. We have the extract that neutralizes Valley Fever. Intravenous garlic is the most effective treatment for getting rid of it. I've seen nothing but good results treating Valley Fever. Instead of taking an anti-fungal for six months or one year, patients can get rid of their Valley Fever within a few weeks.

I am very grateful to the state of Arizona for giving me the opportunity to practice freely without persecution by the medical authorities for the past 32 years, and for the opportunity to help so many who have few places to turn.

ABRAM BER, MD, MD(H)
Homeopathic Physician
5011 North Granite Reef Road
Scottsdale, Arizona 85250
(480)941-2141

Dennis J. Courtney, MD

McMURRAY, PENNSYLVANIA

Interviewed August 4, 2013

1. **Every good alternative doctor knows that an initial consultation probably can't be accomplished in less than two hours.**

2. **Correcting both deficiencies and toxicities is an essential component of any heath care program.**

3. **Every individual, no matter how compromised or healthy, requires six categories of supplements on a daily basis.**

DR. KONDROT: My good friend, Dr. Dennis Courtney, has his own very popular radio show in western Pennsylvania. Please share a little bit about your medical background and how you made the transition to having one of the top alternative practices in the United States.

DR. COURTNEY: My initial training in the field of anesthesiology was the first opportunity that I had to be involved in patient care. Putting a patient to sleep for a surgery and then emerging them from the anesthesia back to consciousness once again is truly an art form. The time I spent as an anesthesiologist was quite rewarding, and I look back on that time in my career and am thankful for it. I have often said that the surgical division of medicine does not have the demons and controversy that plague some of the other disciplines. A skilled surgeon will always be required to correct some anatomical anomaly by excising first and reconnecting the excised tissue so that the body part is restored to full function. To enable the surgeon to achieve this outcome, the anesthesiologist adds his skill. After a brief recovery period, the patient is able to return to full function once again. It is for this reason that I refer to the surgical division of medicine as a "clean" science.

Internal medicine and the other medical specialties are something completely different because treating chronic disease means that the patient is never actually better. The patient continues on a medical regimen of pharmaceuticals that never actually comes to a conclusion. How can medicines be expected to resolve a medical problem when all the drugs being used are only meant to control the symptoms of the disease but not the disease itself? This symptomatic approach to the treatment of disease perpetuates a cycle that never really ends and frustrates doctors and patients alike, leading to what I refer to as "dirty medicine." You would think that a primary care physician would jump at the opportunity to take another approach to disease, an approach that actually has at its core the resolution of a disease rather than its symptoms.

DR. KONDROT: So what sparked your interest in pursuing alternative medicine and ultimately leaving the anesthesia profession?

DR. COURTNEY: It was the mid-'90s and all was going well with my anesthesia work when I met lay people who began to talk about certain medical treatments that I had not heard about. One in partic-

ular that they said they were pursuing was able to remove plaque from the inside of arteries and was called chelation therapy. I had never heard of the term "chelation" before and when I was told that it was an IV therapy that was able to "dissolve" plaque on the inside of the arteries, I responded by telling them that they obviously must be mistaken because, as a doctor, I had never heard of such a thing. At that point, besides telling me about chelation therapy and how it works, they went one step further and gave me information that I could study on the subject. This information was written by other medical professionals, and it was fully referenced with multiple sources of articles and textbooks. It was clear that they were right, and that there was a therapy that could "dissolve" plaque on the inside of arteries. It was at this point that I frantically searched my wall full of medical books to find some corroboration in the medical literature. After an extensive search, I concluded that there was not one mention in any of the books that chelation therapy even existed. How could it be that such a seemingly important and beneficial treatment, with limitless potential to help those afflicted with cardiovascular disease and plaque formation, didn't make it into even one of those books?

I knew the answer to my rhetorical question. The absence was not by accident or oversight but instead by conscious intent to omit and ignore. Now, almost 20 years later, I have file cabinets full of patient charts that continue to confirm the assertions made by those chelation enthusiasts from the mid-'90s, and the number of satisfied patients continues to grow annually.

DR. KONDROT: Well, Dr. Courtney, it appears that chelation therapy was your introduction to the realm of alternative medicine, but how did your philosophical approach to treating patients alternatively evolve?

DR. COURTNEY: In over 17 years of practicing integrated medicine, I have had the honor of improving the health of thousands of patients. Some of those patients were very energetic and enthusiastic and had admirable lifestyles and eating habits in an attempt to optimize their health. At the other end of the spectrum were those with chronic disease and compromised abilities due to many years of neglect and lifestyle choices that led to the deterioration of their health. In this group, there were those with serious advanced disease who had decreased ability to walk without pain or shortness of breath. Still another group of patients in this category were those who could be called the "walking wounded." These patients are probably the most difficult to work with because they insist that they feel great even when confronted with evidence to the contrary. With all patients, my hope is to enter into a partnership that will allow them to follow a plan to achieve optimal health.

As a physician, my challenge continues to be my ability to successfully arouse the interest level in patients so that they will "buy into" this partnering concept no matter what their level of health happens to be. Not only must the message I convey to patients be appealing and accurate, it must be clearly explained so that, if it is followed, it will yield the results that were promised. To reach the point where a true partnership can be formed between doctor and patient, two objectives must be accomplished.

1. Present the message at the first meeting so that the patient can actually feel enthusiasm beginning to build so that, by the conclusion of the encounter, he or she leaves my office with a sense of excitement about our plan.

2. The health message itself must be simple and easily understood.

1. Every good alternative doctor knows that an initial consultation probably can't be accomplished in less than two hours.

With respect to the first of these objectives, the patient must be made to feel that only he or she really matters to me. This becomes apparent when the patient notices that the doctor *never looks at his watch*. This demonstrates a commitment that the doctor is going to make to listen intently to what the patients say about themselves in response to the doctor's questions. Wise mentors of mine were quick to point out that patients will tell you what is wrong with them. I now know no truer words have ever been spoken. This encounter takes considerable time and every good alternative doctor knows that an initial consultation probably can't be accomplished in less than two hours.

The next thing to remember is to keep it simple. If the doctor gets carried away with lofty concepts and discussing controversial therapies on this first visit, it may very well be the last time that he will see that patient. Keeping it simple is equally beneficial with those patients who are well informed on the subject of their health. It was out of this awareness that that I developed "the treatment tripod." After the listening phase is over, and it's time for me to take control of the conversation, my "go to" message will easily characterize the doctor-patient relationship and the treatment that follows.

DR. KONDROT: It's interesting that your transition occurred right around my transition in the mid-'90s. That's when I gradually phased out of my ophthalmic surgical practice and made that transition into alternative treatments that I feel are truly helping patients in a much more profound manner. Tell us more about this treatment tripod.

DR. COURTNEY: The "treatment tripod" can be conceptualized as the foundation for improving health. Every program needs a beginning — a start-up point

— and, as I previously stated, requires a simple message. The "treatment tripod" provides that starting point and that message. It is the firm foundation that will be built upon as the initial treatment objectives are attained.

I look at the tripod as though they are the legs of a three-legged stool. Every leg depends on the other two to provide necessary support and stability. If one leg is uneven or wobbly, the entire structure crashes. The three legs of this tripod:

1. Deficiency States - Diagnosis and Correction

2. Toxic States - Diagnosis and Correction

3. Perfusion - Adequate optimal blood flow to all tissues that will facilitate the ability to correct the other two states

2. Correcting both deficiencies and toxicities is an essential component of any heath care program.

The general observations that I should make about the treatment tripod are that two of the three legs of the stool have been the bedrock of integrative medicine for at least a half century. It should be no surprise to clinicians and patients alike that correcting both deficiencies and toxicities is an essential component of a heath care program. I would like to share with you, however, what I feel are some distinct approaches that I use to accomplish this. I share my view with all of my colleagues and patients and remain available for their scrutiny of my approach.

The third leg of the stool, "Perfusion of the tissues," I feel is not pursued by the integrative professional medical community nearly enough to allow for the other two legs on the tripod to be optimal. I would like to see increased interest in developing optimal perfusion of the tissues. So we will discuss each of the legs of the tripod or stool and include the commentary that will allow you to decide if we can improve upon how these tasks will be achieved.

The first leg of the tripod refers to deficiency states that develop within the human body. Over the course of a lifetime, various and multiple nutrients, which are required for optimal cell function, are just not supplied in the correct amount. Even in the case of those who eat a well-balanced diet, their diets do not supply adequate levels of all the vital nutrients due to the fact that the soil where the foods are grown is depleted. Due to this soil depletion, foods, no matter how wonderful they appear, don't contain sufficient nutrients to supply the body with its needs. Consequently, you must supplement with the appropriate vitamins and minerals on a daily basis if the enzyme systems of the body are to function optimally. This has led to one of the most frequently asked questions that I get from patients, which is, "Doc, what supplements should I take? Just tell me what to take and I'll do it." This is an important question asked of all physicians by patients.

My answer to the question until just a few years ago was to never really name a special product. To be honest I wasn't impressed by any of them. The vast majority of vitamins are synthetic. Just read the label on the vitamin bottle that you use. The ingredients are synthetic. I just don't like synthetic anything. On the other hand, the whole food version of vitamins never lists their ingredients other than the foods they come from. In that case there is just no way to standardize the content. Instead of answering the question about what supplements to take directly, it has been my practice to answer this way:

3. Every individual no matter how compromised or healthy has six categories of supplements that they require on a daily basis.

As you may suspect it usually requires that the individual purchase six separate products to meet the physiological benefits of adequate supplementation. The categories are:

Category One: A Good Multivitamin

As mentioned, multivitamins are either synthetic or whole foods derived. The best advice to give patients is to go with a company with a good and well-respected reputation.

Category Two: Macro Minerals

This category refers to the daily intake of sodium, potassium, calcium, and magnesium. These four elements must be represented in large quantities every single day. It's possible to get a good multivitamin with those four already in it, but sometimes it requires a second supplement to be taken all by itself.

Category Three: Trace Minerals

There are many micro minerals which require daily replacement in the human body. These trace minerals are required to complete a multitude of enzymatic reactions. You need every one of these special molecules to promote bio-chemical reactions. If they are not provided, the body will have to perform a work around in order to complete the reaction, and this is much less efficient than it would have been with the specific micro mineral required.

Category Four: Essential Fats

This category is often misunderstood. For our purposes, let's just say that the Omega 3 and Omega 6 fatty acids that the body requires must be supplied daily in specific amounts and that we cannot rely on food to supply them. It should also be mentioned that the daily consumption of fish oil does not provide the correct fatty acids either. What is more important is to be clear that taking fish oil can be hazardous to your health. The correct oils on the Omega 6 side of the ledger as a category are represented by safflower oil and primrose oil. On the Omega 3 side the oil category is represented by flax seed and chia oil. The final point to make about fatty acids is that it has been scientifically determined that the proper ratio of these fatty acids is four to one Omega 6 to Omega 3.

Category Five: The Enzymes

To properly digest the foods that you eat you will need to add enzymes to your supplemental regime. Natural enzymes are usually destroyed through heating and cooking. You will need to take lipases (for fats), protease (for proteins), and amylase (for carbohydrates).

Category Six: Antioxidants

There are many different biochemical reactions in the human body that generate reactive oxygen species (ROS), which have deleterious consequences at the membrane level of the cell. To be able to limit the potential harm that can be caused by this oxidative damage, a healthy daily dose of antioxidants is recommended.

After so many years of not recommending any supplement by name, I have finally become comfortable with doing so. The reason that this is now possible is that a new category of supplementation is available that is neither synthetic nor whole food. The newer products on the market are referred to as Bio-Algae Concentrates (BAC). With these newer products it is now possible to get all six categories of supplements in one product.

DR. KONDROT: What I like about the treatment tripod is that if you think about a tripod, you cannot wobble it if the three legs are firm. Dr. Courtney's treatment tripod is one way for you to understand your problem and regain your health. You have explained the first leg of the tripod — deficiency.

DR. COURTNEY: Now, let's turn our attention to the second leg of the tripod, the toxicity states of the human body. As was the case with deficiencies interfering with cellular function, especially when those deficiencies have accrued over a lifetime, the same can be said about toxic substances. Toxic substances gain access through all routes of penetration: air, water, food, chemicals, skin exposure, and so on year after year. These substances interfere with a multitude of cellular reactions that inhibit the organ or body tissue involved, and eventually it functions sub optimally and, finally, not at all. Alternative doctors have done well in recognizing the deleterious effects of these toxic substances and have done a good job in assisting the body to eliminate them.

When it comes to clearing toxic substances, one of the most basic things to do is to purge these substances though cleanses. Once or twice a year, use such things as colon/liver cleanses, colon cleanses, gall bladder cleanses. All are important to "scrub up" the cellular waste products surrounding the vital organs of the GI system. These organs tend to get "gummed up" with more toxic substances than any others.

Another level of toxic burden involves heavy metal toxicity. Some form of testing should be employed to determine which metals are present and the amount of those metals which are detected. Two forms of testing for heavy metals are not very helpful. Blood testing is rarely helpful because toxic metals are rarely found in the blood. Chronic heavy metal exposure places metals deep within the body tissues, and they must be pulled into the blood through a provocative chelating agent so that the metal can be identified. Hair testing is also a problem, even though it is very commonly used as a screening tool. There are so many inaccuracies in hair testing that I would never consider doing it.

The most accurate heavy metal testing requires having the patient take a chelating agent and then testing for metals by analyzing the patient's urine that has been collected over a 24-hour period. I have used provocative testing for many years and have become comfortable with using prescription level chelating agents to remove metals. I now question the use of these harsh chemical substances to eliminate heavy metals from the body. I prefer the approach of a brilliant biochemist, Dr. Patricia Kane. She has developed a technique using natural non-toxic substances to remove the heavy metal burden without using toxic pharmaceutical substances.

Let us now turn our attention to the

third leg of the tripod, which refers to optimal perfusion of all tissues in the human body. It is my assertion that as well as the integrative medical community has done with correcting deficiencies and toxicities of their patients, they have done poorly with improving perfusion of all the organs of the human body by optimizing the patient's cardiovascular system. To take that one step further: if you don't take the time to optimize perfusion, you really can't ever correct the deficiencies and toxicities. It stands to reason that you must provide a blood supply to an area in order to bring nutrients to it and, likewise, if you expect to remove toxic substances and heavy metals, there must be a well-developed blood flow from the region to carry the offensive substance to the organs of elimination.

It just happens that treating cardiovascular disease effectively has as one of its benefits the ability to maximize perfusion to all areas of the body while interrupting a degenerative pathological process that tops the list as the leading cause of death in this country. As a direct result of maximizing perfusion to the tissues, all organs of the body receive optimal blood flow, which then supports optimal cellular function.

There are four steps to reversing cardiovascular disease and in the process maximizing perfusion to the tissues.

1. Correct inflammation risk factors.

2. Remove cardiovascular plaque.

3. Maximize new blood vessel formation through ECP.

4. Dissolve clots.

Correction of Inflammation Risk Factors

The endothelial lining of the heart and blood vessels is continually under assault in men over the age of 18 and in women in their post-menopausal years. This assault takes the form of an irritation and inflammation of both structures due to substances found in the blood that come into contact with this lining 24 hours a day, 7 days a week, 365 days a year. These elements that are found in everybody's blood have to be within certain parameters of normalcy. If their levels move outside of these normal ranges, they have the potential to irritate, inflame, and damage the lining of blood vessels.

The first thing that must be done is to obtain a laboratory analysis of the blood to determine the 13 inflammatory risk factors. I consider them to be 13 potential fires that stoke the flames that literally could be rated as three alarm blazes going on throughout the body. It is certainly unusual, if not downright embarrassing, that these tests are never ordered by doctors. The reason that doctors don't order these tests is because there is no medicine to correct 12 of the 13 markers. They only have medicine to treat one of them. So, doctors don't want to alarm a patient without providing a solution for the problem. Doctors understandably don't order the blood tests at all.

Integrative doctors have an advantage over conventional doctors in that we do not need to use a medicine to correct the abnormally elevated inflammation marker. Instead, through the use of minerals, vitamins, herbs, or other modalities, we are able to extinguish all 13 inflammation factors and completely put out the fire. We will save the discussion about these 13 blood tests for another day. Let's now discuss perfusion maneuver number two: remove plaque.

Remove Cardiovascular Plaque

The second of the four components to optimize the perfusion of the heart and blood vessels is the removal of arterial plaque. It is the damage done to the lining of the heart and blood vessels by inflammation that leads to the endless deposition of plaque. Most integrative doctor's chelation therapy does remove plaque. I have file cabinets filled with the charts of patients that have had that plaque dissolved through the use of a substance called EDTA. Whether it is administered orally, intravenously, or rectally is a professional choice. Whether it is to be used at all is a medical necessity.

Maximize New Blood Vessel Formation through ECP

The third component of increasing perfusion is to increase the actual number of blood vessels able to carry blood throughout the body by a procedure known as ECP, which is an acronym for External Counter Pulsation. Of all the items I've mentioned so far that increase blood flow through the human body, none works as well as ECP. ECP is an FDA approved, insurance covered procedure that consists of 35 treatments that are given one hour a day, five days a week for seven weeks using a special device. The procedure consists of leg and hip compression with large inflatable cuffs, which perform the compression maneuvers in synchronicity with the heart, moving large volumes of blood from the hips and lower extremities into the central circulation above the waist assailing all organs of the upper torso rhythmically with each heartbeat. Through a hormonal mechanism, brand new blood vessels are created establishing augmented perfusion to all organs.

Dissolve Clots

The final component of the plan to improve perfusion is to dissolve clots. These clots are generated around the periphery of plaque formation due to the oozing of blood from the damaged lining of arteries. They may grow to substantial size and have the potential to become dislodged and abruptly occlude arteries downstream. When the artery occluded is in the heart, the event is called a heart attack. When the artery occluded is in the brain, the event is called a stroke. When the event occurs in any other organ, it is called an infarct.

The conventional medical community has no mild clot busting medicine available. The integrative medical community has the ability to gently dissolve clots through a category of non-prescription substances known as the Kinases. The two best known of this group of clot busting substances are Nattokinase and Boluoke Lumbrokinase.

DR. KONDROT: I'm beginning to understand your treatment tripod, but what are some of your favorite ways of evaluating patients? Where do you begin? Tell me a little bit about your approach.

DR. COURTNEY: With respect with what happens when someone first meets me, I need information. I already know that the diseases they're seeing me for are going to involve deficiencies and toxicities. This is no surprise. These people are starved for nutrition and don't have the right components to their nutrient profile, and they're loaded with toxicities.

I start with the heart. I do a major workup for the cardiovascular system to know how I can get this heart in play. It's where I begin and where I end. It's being able to use the deficiency corrections and toxicity removals with a higher level of efficiency because I've already made the correction to the system that's moving things around.

....

DENNIS J. COURTNEY, MD
The Courtney Medical Group
3075 Washington Road
McMurray, PA 15317
(724)942-3002
www.djcmd.com
info@DJCMD.com

Gabriel Cousens MD, MD(H)

PATAGONIA, ARIZONA

Interviewed July 7, 2013

1. In three weeks, 61% of Type 2 non-insulin-dependent diabetics are healed. Healed means their blood sugar is less than 100 with no insulin or other diabetes medications.

2. The second level of healing means to live a life that's going to give you steady enduring radiant health at any age, at any time of the day, and any time of the year.

DR. KONDROT: Gabriel Cousens, who is a medical doctor, a doctor of Homeopathy, a Diplomat of the American Board of Integrative Holistic Medicine, a Diplomat of Ayurveda, a Doctor of Divinity, a Rabbi, a Native American Sundancer, and acknowledged yogi, who's a member of the Arizona Homeopathic and Integrative Medical Association. He is the founder of the Tree of Life Center, and he has written several books.

DR. COUSENS: Actually, it's ten books.

DR. KONDROT: My apologies for not being up to speed on that. I know that one of the books, *The Rainbow Green Live-Food Cuisine*, is one of my favorites. I have it in my office, and I often refer to it. I really admire you for the work you're doing in lighting the fire under people to tell them that there is a way to achieve health and treat diabetes naturally.

Please tell about your medical background and how your practice evolved to incorporate more of the holistic approach?

DR. COUSENS: I need to start when I was four years old when I announced to my parents that I wanted to be a doctor. I didn't know what a doctor was, and nobody in my family had ever been a doctor. That's the background. It was like a very early program. I pursued it in high school. In the '50s, I built a heart-lung machine. This was before they were used in hospitals. I won the state science fair prize with that invention.

Then I went to Amherst College in Massachusetts, one of the top small colleges in the country. There, I built another heart-lung machine and did other research including publishing my first paper in the *Biochemical & Biophysics Research Communication Journal*. I was also the captain of an undefeated Amherst College football team and inducted into the National Football Hall of Fame as a scholar athlete.

I majored in biochemistry at Amherst College and then went to Columbia Medical School in New York City. I found myself fascinated more with internal medicine, even though I was heavily pushed toward orthopedics for a variety of reasons. I ended up going into holistic psychiatry and family therapy. However, when I got out of medical school and finished my psychiatry residency, I realized that the mind and the body were really connected. So in 1973, 40 years ago, I began combining the mind and body in my approach in what people now call "holistic medicine."

Through the lens of my biochemistry background and my holistic medical and spiritual background, I began observing that many people had blood sugar imbalances and a variety of chronic diseases. This was before the terms "holistic medicine" and "integrative medicine" were anything people really knew about.

What I did know, as a third-year medical student at Columbia, was that conventional medicine did not have any clue about how to heal disease. It was very clear to me. They also did not know how to prevent disease. I was very aware that conventional medicine did not really understand what was going on, and, therefore, was quite unsuccessful. That's how I became interested in psychiatry; I saw the mind as a key player in overall health.

After my psychiatry residency, I studied a variety of naturopathic medicine areas. I studied herbalism; I studied homeopathy with a four-year course; I studied acupuncture and Chinese herbs and took the UCLA acupuncture course for doctors and graduated from that. I was a natural candidate for the Arizona Homeopathic and Integrative Medicine Association, under which I was licensed in 1987. This board was a perfect design for me to practice optimal holistic medicine.

I also do a lot of work with what we call orthomolecular medicine and orthomolecular psychiatry, and I combined them in a total holistic approach. If I see a family, I may do family therapy or individual work. I assess globally how to approach the situation with a whole variety of tools, from individual psychotherapy to family therapy to couple therapy. That's how my practice evolved to include a holistic evaluation of the individual person.

The first 20 years of my practice, in California, focused on developing a holistic approach. I moved to Arizona in 1987 when the homeopathic license was available. It was very clear that this was an optimal situation for practicing the highest level of holistic medicine with colleagues who really understood what it was about. My experience with the holistic, homeopathic doctors who are licensed that way is that they are the most sophisticated doctors I have met in the whole country, really in the whole world. It is really an honor to be part of the Arizona Homeopathic and Integrative Medicine Association.

The other approach I added is that I saw that healing needed to be more global. When I was in Petaluma, California, you could tell people to improve their diets or do other things for their health, but they didn't have the background to hold to a program so easily.

I created the Tree of Life Center US where I work with clients in a surround-around setting to support their total holistic healing. People can come and learn how to prepare organic and plant-source, only live food. I can train them how to relate as couples within a total lifestyle so they can continue the surround-around experience after they leave. That's the model I've been using at

the Tree of Life Center in Patagonia, Arizona, since 1993. We have 181 acres where people come and stay and live the lifestyle. For three days, a few weeks, or even months, they get a taste of a new way of living. It's more experiential and, therefore, supports a total holistic health transition.

I'm very happy because I'm also now living the holistic lifestyle. We're out in the country. Patagonia, as you may know, has 800 people. We're up in the mountains at 4,000 feet elevation. We have the fourth cleanest air in the United States. Everything I write about in my books, I'm doing. That's the overview. It has to be good for everyone, so I also have to do it.

DR. KONDROT: Your center is not only educational but it's experiential. People actually live the holistic life they need to help regain their health. I want you to talk about some of your books. I also want you to share your findings that most cases of Type 2 Diabetes can be treated successfully by looking very carefully at diet and lifestyle changes and getting off the harmful petrochemicals that people are taking to regulate their blood sugar.

1. In three weeks, 61% of Type 2 non-insulin-dependent diabetics are healed. Healed means blood sugar is less than 100 with no insulin or other diabetes medications.

DR. COUSENS: My latest book is called *There is a Cure for Diabetes.* I have a 21-day program for healing both diabetes and transitioning to optimal health. During the program, we put the residents on a special diet that's moderately low carbohydrate, 100% live food. It's completely plant-source only. In three weeks, 61% of Type 2 non-insulin-dependent diabetics are healed. Healed means their blood sugar is less than 100 without insulin or other diabetes medications. Twenty-four percent of Type 2 insulin-dependent diabetics are off all insulin, all medications, and have a blood sugar less than 100. Amazingly, 21% of the Type 1 diabetics, who are supposedly totally incurable, were healed in three weeks, off all insulin or oral diabetic medications with a blood sugar less than 100.

We got some pretty good results. No one in the world has gotten anything close to that.

Again, it's something that I can do here in Arizona in a way that is unfettered, so I can give the highest level of healthcare to people.

DR. KONDROT: What's the secret to your success? Diabetes is becoming a major problem in our country. The incidence is increasing.

DR. COUSENS: It's a pandemic around the world.

DR. KONDROT: It's leading to two to four times increased rates in heart disease, vascular disease, eye disease, and other endocrine problems.

DR. COUSENS: Sugar is the food choice of cancer cells. It increases the incidences of cancer and heart disease three to fourfold. Three-quarters of people with diabetes die of heart disease. Twenty to fifty percent develop end stage kidney disease. Seventy percent develop neuropathy, and 85% of diabetics develop retinopathy. Alzheimer's is doubled and depression is increased three to fourfold. It's a disaster. The good news is that not only can diabetes be reversed and cured, but these diabetes degenerative syndromes can be reversed even including blindness.

The secret to our success is pretty simple. We do a moderate to low healthy carbohydrate diet that's 25% to 35% complex carbohydrates. This is the healing diet. It's comprised of 25% to 35% complex carbohydrates, meaning leafy greens, sprouts and all the vegetables. We do 25% to 45% plant-based fats and 10% to 25% plant-based protein. It is a key, teaching that the diet needs to be individualized to a person's genetic constitution to have maximum benefit. Seventy-five percent of the population needs a higher protein diet and 25% need a lower protein diet. The other thing that's a key element for healing is 100% live food. These two things combined with eating organic are the foundation of my healing system that works not only for diabetes, but almost all major chronic diseases. This is what I call phase 1.0. Then we add meditation and yoga. We get people walking and exercising. We monitor them four times a day and take their blood sugars, but the diet is the key factor.

After the initial round of one week of green juice fasting, we add herbs that increase the function of the pancreas and the total system around insulin production. Once a client is healed, and they stay that way for three months, we go to a second level of diet, or phase 1.5.

The book *Rainbow Green Live-Food Cuisine* describes phase 1 and phase 1.5. The healing diet is phase 1. Then we add cherries, berries, grains, beans, and things like that, and up to 20% cooked food, if they choose, when they have gone three months with a blood sugar less than 100 and no medications. This has been very successful.

I have initiated diabetes prevention programs in 16 different countries. We're spreading this information around the world because it's a worldwide pandemic. It's very simple. It means eliminating white flour, white sugar, and junk food. These so called food items are the driving force behind the pandemic of diabetes.

When we look at the emergence of diabetes on a worldwide basis, the Pima Indians, who live in southern Arizona, are a good example. They had one case in 1920. Now, 90% of the Pima Indians have diabetes. What's the difference? It's called white sugar.

It's not that complex. Every medical school will tell you, "You shouldn't have sugar." That's not what we say. We say, "You shouldn't have *any* sugar." That's the difference. It's the intensity of the approach that makes the difference in the Dr. Cousens Diabetes Recovery Program. The live food makes the difference. There are some healing factors to the live food that really accelerate the process.

My Diabetes Recovery Program is an intense three-week healing process. The advantage of this short time is that people become very inspired by their rapidly visible positive results and become committed to the diet. After that, I do use other things like homeopathics, but the whole idea is that diet, moderate exercise, and adequate sleep are the keys. It works. I've been doing this for about seven years.

Included in the 21-Day Transformation Program is our Conscious Eating Program that empowers people to prepare tasty, low-glycemic live foods. They really know how to prepare the food when they leave. I include a four-day psycho-spiritual course in the 21-Day Program as well. It is important to address the psycho-spiritual issues because diabetes involves that as well. This 21-day synergy helps them to really make the breakthrough. When people are successful, they become more motivated.

Having success in three weeks is really good. For Type I diabetics, in three weeks, there's a 67% drop in the insulin need for those people who didn't get cured. Thirty-one percent of the Type I diabetics were able to go off all insulin and 21% were healed. These are very clear results.

In the Type II diabetes results from my book, I present a comprehensive theory of

Type II diabetes and how to heal it. Type II diabetes is an epigenetic downgrade that affects what we call lepton and insulin hormonal imbalance. Epigenetic means that the genetic expression has been modified due to external factors. This epigenetic downgrade is set off by a diet high in white sugar, white flour, junk food, pesticides, herbicides, and so forth. It's actually quite simple. Our program upgrades the epigenetic program back to normal.

DR. KONDROT: So a diabetic needs to shift his or her diet more towards 100% live food, greens, complex carbohydrates and eliminate bad elements, which are primarily white flour, white sugar, and junk food. This is similar to the approach I use at my wellness center. Dr. Cousins, your approach not only works with Type II diabetes but also with many other conditions. I wonder if you could describe that.

2. The second level of healing means to live a life that's going to give you steady enduring radiant health at any age, at any time of the day and any time of the year.

DR. COUSENS: I'm really happy because in a global way, we're not treating disease. In a global way, I'm creating enduring global radiant health. That's the model. I have my prevention program activated in 16 different countries at this point.

The first stage of enduring radiant health is making a mental shift so that you really begin to connect, not only with diet, but with a total holistic lifestyle, including some spiritual connection.

When people come for treatment, whether they're here for a day, a week, three weeks, or three months, it is about helping them shift their paradigm in terms of allowing that they are not their disease.

All kinds of chronic diseases are healed at the Tree of Life Center US. I have extremely good success, about 95%, with chronic fatigue, which is also a major plague today and with chronic fibromyalgia with about 95% of people healing from the syndrome. I also have about a 95% success rate with high blood pressure in one to three weeks.

I also do a lot of work with depression. I have a book called *Depression-Free for Life*. I heal it naturally by getting people off all their medications, rebuilding their neurotransmitter systems, and helping them maintain a healthy life. Healing really happens across the board for pretty much all chronic disease.

I do very little treatment of cancer and AIDS. Those are two areas I stay away from, but with everything else the same basic principles apply.

In addition to the lifestyle, exercise, meditation, and opening up to who you are in your life, we give special nutrients, both herbs and homeopathy. I use a full range of Chinese herbs, Ayurvedic herbs, and American herbs as well as homeopathy. I do homeopathy with every client. This comprehensive program is tailored to each person's individual needs.

One of the key mistakes people make in diet is they think the same diet is good for everyone. In my book, *Conscious Eating,* which I wrote in 1990 and rewrote in 2000, I make the point that we have to individualize diet according to our unique constitutions. We help people find their unique constitution and eat accordingly. Along with that their lifestyle has to be re-organized to their unique constitution.

Besides the individual, I also look at the relationship aspect because relationship plays a huge role in somebody's health. There was a study in the 1930s in England that showed that the quality of health a person had, correlated specifically with how their family was doing. It's called the Pioneer Study and was a ten-year study, interrupted by World War II.

The point is we are significantly affected by our family associations. Including this aspect of wellness is a very global approach on the physical and emotional level as well as the family level. Then, of course, there is the spiritual level. It's that global approach that brings the results into the 90% and 95% success rates for most chronic degenerative diseases. This is the first stage of healing.

The second stage is learning how to go to enduring radiant health. My age is 70. When I was 60, I did 601 pushups. At the age of 70, without any practice, I did 300 pushups, but I have nothing impeding me. All my football injuries are gone including a torn cartilage in my left knee and a torn rotator cuff in my right shoulder, all of which healed without surgery. There is what I call a free flow in the physical body. That means I can sit for hours in full lotus. I can do whatever I need to physically. I have no physical impediments.

What I am talking about is the meaning of enduring, radiant health. That's the next level. Your mind is working right. Your body is working right, and this can be true at any age. When Moshe Rabbeinu (Moses) left his body at 120, it's said that his eyes were fine, and his vision had not degenerated, and he had no loss of vitality.

That's the model of enduring radiant health that we have today and that I'm helping people go toward. The first level is to clear up all the imbalances. The second level is live a life that's going to give you that steady enduring radiant health at any age at any time of the day and any time of the year.

DR. KONDROT: I have to admire a physician like you who truly walks the talk. I was actually kind of shocked when you told me your age is 70 because I thought you were much younger.

DR. COUSENS: At a certain level, I've cracked the code of how one does it. That's the second level, but that's not what I deal with in the first level. The first level is to clear up the disease and get yourself in balance. Then it's the second level where one moves to enduring, radiant health. That is the stage I am promoting by my own living example. I'm happily married. I have three grandchildren. People say when they're old, "I wish I had the energy I had when I was 20, but the wisdom of when I'm 70." You've probably heard that. With our program, you *have* the energy of a 20-year-old and the wisdom of a 70-year-old. It's a great combination, and it is a lot of fun.

DR. KONDROT: When somebody comes to your center, what type of evaluation do you perform? How do you determine what type of program they're going to need?

DR. COUSENS: I do a three-day evaluation. I do a variety of in-house tests, including a three to five hour glucose tolerance test. I do a lot of work with what I call the diabetes degenerative syndrome, which means blood sugar spiking, pre-diabetes, hypoglycemia, and then diabetes. I'm looking to see the pattern. A great many people have disorganization in their glucose metabolism. That's one of the things I specialize in.

Then I spend approximately two and a half or three hours per person in the initial visit. The second visit is in two to three months for one and a half to two hours. I offer the Rolls Royce of holistic work-ups. It's just my style. I want to give people complete attention and time. I'll typically spend the whole morning with somebody because I want to look at every-thing and put the whole picture together before I give them a detailed plan.

People need to come for at least three days to get organized and to be part of the lifestyle. At the end of that, I give them the full work-up. It's very traditional in that it is very thoughtful and focused. This is the way physicians, such as Moses Maimonides in the 12th Century and Paracelsus several centuries later, have worked.

Then I may see the patient two to three months later, but if all is going well and they're progressing well, then in six months. In other words, they do the work. We do phone call follow-ups to monitor them on a monthly or bimonthly basis. People have come to my program from over 112 nations.

The second aspect of the healing process is empowerment training. I have courses on how to prepare the food. I have a course called the Zero Point, which is a self-guided spiritual psycho-therapy technique they do on them-selves. I have fasting, detox, and spiritual fasting retreats. I offer training in organic farming, so that people may be inspired to grow their own food.

Over a year, people become very empowered to live a holistic lifestyle. You can't do it all at once. It takes a little time. Honestly, it's not for everybody. We in the holistic field have to recognize that not everybody is that interested in actually changing themselves. This approach only works for people who really want to change themselves and to transition into a higher quality of total life in terms of how their relationship and mind/body/spirit is. It is for people who want to be fully vibrant, turned-on people. That's what we're going for.

DR. KONDROT: It's so different from traditional Western tradition where the doctor will spend five minutes with you, write out a prescription, and say, "Come back in a week." The person doesn't get any better. They get more ill, and there's no return to wellness and health.

DR. COUSENS: That's not part of my model. When I saw it in medical school, I said, "I can't do that; it is not a working model."

DR. KONDROT: Gabriel, please share with us a little bit about your vision for improving the health of the world.

DR. COUSENS: I wanted to start with an understanding that not everybody in the world sees allopathic medicine as we see it in the United States. In my work with diabetes and general health that I'm doing in about 16 different countries, there is a much greater perception of how important it is to return to the natural way.

I'm working in Africa — in Ethiopia, Ghana, Cameroon, and Nigeria — and in Israel, Taiwan, Singapore, Bali, Papua, New Guinea, Argentina, Peru, Mexico, Nicaragua, and a lot of different places. People in these countries are not that removed from the natural way.

The first step is to begin to move back into the natural way. What does that mean? It means eating homegrown, organic, natural foods. When we go that way, we move away from fast food, white flour, white sugar, and junk food. Live according to the cycles of life and cycles of the day. It's dramatic.

I remember being in Ghana. I have established a Cousens Health Center there for all the kids. We put in two wells to give them fresh water. We were having a rally and the local king hosting me said, "What we want to drink is water. We don't need soft drinks. Throw away your soft drinks. Go back to water, soft drinks are poison." He's completely correct. When you look at soft drinks, white sugar, white flour, and junk food, you see that it has been a complete disaster for health worldwide. It makes money for some people, but it's a worldwide disaster.

One finds that people around the world know this. When we step out of the industrial, corporate, pharmaceutical world of the United States, one sees a natural way of life that we are trying to return to with our holistic medicine approaches. In other countries, people know about herbal cures and natural remedies and the natural way to live in the world.

My input as I work at national governmental levels is to encourage them to go back to their natural ways. Everybody knows them because they're only one or two generations removed.

Grow locally. Food grown locally is actually cheaper, has more nutrients, is fresher, and is easier to obtain. We actually have a master's program in veganic farming here at the Tree of Life Center US. It's from our Tree of Life Foundation, which is a nonprofit corporation.

We have a master's program in live food nutrition as well. We're training people to go to these countries and teach. To me, it's about re-educating people back to the natural ways. It seems redundant or like an oxymoron, but it isn't. When people come from the United States and they have the training to say, "Go back to your natural ways," people have permission to actually do that. That's probably the most important outcome of our work internationally.

In Papua, New Guinea, where 40% of the people have diabetes, I addressed the problem. I talked to the representatives and the prime minister. They have no problem with this concept. It's easy. People are aware. We come in with our expertise from the United States and say, "You're right."

I've also addressed the Russian parliament about diabetes. It's the same thing. I say, "Go back to natural ways. Start eating your live food and your plant-based diet. Stay away from white flour, white sugar, and junk food, and you're going to win most of the battle. Have fresh water." We do a lot of work with water purification because that's pretty fundamental.

In some of the countries, like Ethiopia and Papua, New Guinea, we go so far as talking about taxing junk food and soft drinks. The governments say, "We can't afford the health costs." If they know they can save money by keeping people healthy, they're going to be more motivated to tax the things that are hurting their population's health. Many of the governments around the world are willing to go in that direction. To me, it does need to come from the government's direction to go back to healthy ways, as well as from educating the population.

My work includes a lot of educating at the school level. We train people to go into the schools and teach the kids about healthy eating. We have schools in many of these places. We're serving organic, natural, plant-based foods. Kids love it.

We're working at both the school and government levels to create a return to the way a lot of people know about. That's a simple vision, but we don't need an international corporation to send junk food to you and call that food. This is a problem all over the world. People are impressed with advanced technology and give up their natural birthright without even thinking about it.

I have experience with the Native Americans as well. I was at an international priest/priestess/shaman conference. They were serving hot dogs. I asked, "Are hot dogs your indigenous food?" The grandmothers got it. They said, "Let's go back to our natural, organic food." So the grandmothers took over the food preparation.

This is what I'm doing all over the

world. It's a very simple and attainable vision. There is no need to build more hospitals. Just go back to the way you know how to live.

....

GABRIEL COUSENS, MD, MD(H)
(866)394-2520 (US)
(520)394-2520 (International calls)
www.drcousens.com
info@treeoflife.nu
treeoflifefoundation.org
Patagonia, AZ 85624

There Is a Cure for Diabetes (Revised Edition) can be purchased on www.Amazon.com or at bookstores

Lee Cowden, MD, MD(H)

FLOWER MOUND, TEXAS

Interviewed June 16, 2013

1. **Your own voice may be a powerful healing tool.**

2. **Every physical disease is attached to an emotional conflict.**

3. **Lyme disease can mimic 350 or more diseases and can be transmitted many ways, not just from ticks.**

DR. KONDROT: Dr. Lee Cowden is a very prominent alternative and integrative doctor. He's a board certified cardiologist and internist who is internationally known for his knowledge and skill in practicing and teaching in integrative medicine. In fact, he's on the scientific advisory board of the Academy of Comprehensive Integrative Medicine (ACIM). Please give us a little background about yourself and how you went from being a traditional doctor practicing cardiology to becoming a leader in alternative and integrative medicine.

DR. COWDEN: I actually went into the integrative field very early. I was raised in arid West Texas and went to medical school in Houston. I had been in hot and humid Houston for only a couple of months when I started having a lot of nose and sinus allergies. That changed to infective sinusitis, bronchitis, and finally, pneumonia.

I was following the advice given to me by the chairmen of various medical school departments such as Ear, Nose & Throat, Allergy, and finally the Pulmonary department. Following their advice I got progressively worse.

Thank goodness my wife's grandmother came to visit us. She was a schoolteacher and self-taught nutritionist. She took me down to the health food store and got me on some vitamins, minerals, herbs, and a better diet, and I got well fairly quickly. I thought, "My goodness, I need to learn what this woman knows, and I need to take with a grain of salt everything I learned in medical school and training after this."

During the next few years, I spent my spare time reading about integrative medicine. I first learned about orthomolecular medicine and then Western herbology, Eastern herbology, complex homeopathy, classical homeopathy, fixed magnetic therapies, pulse magnetic therapies, photonic therapies, and so on.

DR. KONDROT: It sounds like your introduction to alternative medicine was very similar to mine. I was a very busy ophthalmic surgeon and I developed asthma. Traditional medicines just made me worse. Finally, when I discovered homeopathy and some alternative treatments and they cured my asthma, I said, "I've got to learn and pursue these disciplines to truly help my patients." There are common things in our background.

I remember the last time we spoke you mentioned EVOX to me. Since we talked a couple of months ago, I have since upgraded my ZYTO machine, and I'm beginning to use EVOX in my practice. I think it's a truly remarkable treatment, so I want you to describe it a little bit,

explain why we're interested in it and how it can help people.

1. Your own voice may be a valuable healing tool.

DR. COWDEN: It is a very valuable technology. I consider it to be in the top five tools of all the tools that I use in helping patients. It's a computerized system where the patient speaks into a microphone. The microphone is not recording the words but the frequencies imbedded in their voice. Each frequency that's recorded corresponds to a specific emotion or belief related to the person or event that they're speaking about. After just 15 seconds of speaking a single word repetitively, the computer screen has a display that shows that patient all the different emotions and beliefs that are attached to the person or event that they were speaking about. Just seeing that display can actually start a healing process.

The device goes a step beyond that and converts the voice frequencies of the patient into what's called harmonic frequencies. That is multiples of the frequency of their own voice, and it delivers those harmonic frequencies back into the patient through an electrode that they grasp while they're listening to pleasant music. Literally, their own voice frequencies shake loose from their cells the emotional cellular memory so that they can actually start getting an emotional healing process that often results in a physical healing as well.

DR. KONDROT: The thing that I find interesting is that it's kind of a passive process for the patient. It's not like deep psychotherapy where you have to talk about your pain, your childhood, or anything like that. It works by speaking for ten seconds. It's not really the content or what you're describing; it's just mainly the tones of your voice. The computer then analyzes the deficiencies or irregularities and balances them on a somewhat of a deeper level.

DR. COWDEN: I've seen that as long as patients can visualize the person or event that they're speaking about, they get quite good results. They don't have to visualize it just with sight. They can recall it with sounds, tastes, touch, and smells as well. The key is to be able to conceptualize it, and, as I said, they can be speaking the same word repetitively.

For example, if they were traumatized by a car wreck, they can just say, "Car wreck, car wreck, car wreck," repeatedly and get the same results as if they were describing the car wreck in great detail with words.

The other thing I do with EVOX is to combine it with a process called Recall Healing. Recall Healing is a conglomeration of therapies that originally started with Ryke Hamer in Germany and then was enhanced by Claude Sabbah in France and by Gilbert Renaud and a variety of other practitioners.

2. Every physical disease is attached to an emotional conflict.

The concept is that every physical disease is attached to an emotional conflict, and, if you know the diagnosis, you can figure out what the conflict was that triggered that physical diagnosis. We use the combination of Recall Healing and EVOX together and get amazing results. People who had previously been undergoing psychotherapy or hypnotized frequently for years get more results from EVOX in one session than they got from five or ten years' worth of therapy with a psychologist or hypnotherapist.

DR. KONDROT: I'm beginning to use that in my practice almost routinely for patients who are losing their vision. Sometimes there's an emotional trigger or emotional component. So far, I just find it really fascinating and amazing. I know it works. Some of the patients have almost an immediate shift in their personality and in their outlook on life, which subsequently, because of this change, enables their body to recover and enables other healing processes to take place such as other treatments that I'm doing to help them regain their sight. I'm happy to hear that you feel it's one of the top five therapies that you do in your practice. I know that you do a lot of amazing things in your practice, so when you say that it's in the top five, I know that I've got to continue using it.

Lee, I know you have an interest in detoxification of the body, and you utilize a unique technique that involves a laser. Please tell us why you use this technique and why you feel it's effective.

DR. COWDEN: In 2001, Cyril Smith, PhD, the quantum physicist, came from England to give a talk at the environmental meeting in Dallas. There he met a PhD anatomist from the University of Texas Southwestern Medical School who was doing research on the microanatomy of the acupuncture meridian system and on the effect of photonic therapies or light on the acupuncture meridian system. They collaborated and came up with the concept of passing laser-pointer light through a clear glass vial containing a homeopathic substance onto the acupuncture points, and it did have a pretty dramatic effect.

The quantum physicist went back to England, and the PhD anatomist continued to do some treatment of patients with that approach, but he was actually causing as much harm as good because he was getting such drastic release of toxins from the body due to the effects of the laser. That's when I came along and helped him come up with ways to do that without harming the patients. It took about a year to figure out all the things that needed to be done.

We learned that physical toxins are held in the body because of unresolved emotional conflicts, and if you use the color therapy along with the laser therapy, you could actually get the toxins to come out without such a harsh response. We also learned that you had to use sufficient amounts of drainage remedies and metal binders whenever you do those therapies; otherwise, the patients' detox organs get overloaded.

DR. KONDROT: It's really a remarkable procedure. You use a regular laser pointer that you can buy at Radio Shack and shine it through a vial or glass container of a homeopathic substance and that light is then projected onto a person. It's not necessary that it hits the skin. You can shine it right through the clothes.

DR. COWDEN: That's right. The patient can be fully clothed. If they have shoes on, they need to take the shoes off, but they can leave their socks on.

We've learned that the most important places to shine the light are on the soles of the feet, the palms of the hands, and the ears, but we also usually shine it on the entire front of the body and the entire back of the body as well. The toxins do come floating out. It's my estimate that the toxins come out about 20 times faster than the next closest competitive technique.

Metals don't come out completely in that first 25 hours, but most non-metallic substances do come out of the body almost completely in 25 hours by energetic testing. Metals start coming out and continue to come out over a period of a few weeks to months after that. That's why it's so important to give the homeopathic drops after that or the heavy-metal binding agents and the drainage remedies. Patients also have to drink plenty of water.

We have found that the patients can neutralize their therapy if they are exposed to a strong electromagnetic field or by being around the chemical that they were trying to detoxify from. If they're trying to detoxify from mercury, we have them avoid eating fish or taking fish oil capsules for 25 hours, and that usually allows them to clear the toxin more efficiently.

DR. KONDROT: This treatment almost sounds like it's too good to be true. It's such a simple technique, and there are no intravenous injections or harmful chemicals being administered. It's just a laser light application.

DR. COWDEN: The doctors who have added it to their practice are continually amazed as I am about how much improvement a patient can get in a very short period of time using this approach.

Years ago, I also noted what I call an energetic autoimmunity. That means patients showed that they were sensitive to hormones and neurotransmitters that were in their own bodies but also showed that they needed those things. They needed them but couldn't tolerate them. When we did laser detox sessions, the patients actually were able to have improvement of the hormonal and neurotransmitter function.

For example, I had a woman who had severe insomnia and never slept more than about three or four hours at a time at night for about ten years. She had tried all kinds of natural and pharmaceutical things with not much success. When we did the energetic evaluation on her, we found that she had an energetic autoimmunity to serotonin and GABA. Those are the two primary neurotransmitters involving sleep. Those appeared to have an autoimmune reaction because of two pesticides in her system.

We made up a homeopathic vial of the two pesticides and a homeopathic vial of GABA and serotonin and did a laser treatment with those four items. That night she slept ten hours without any assistance and continued to sleep eight hours a night after that for months on end until I lost contact with her. I know that it does some amazing things, which don't even seem completely understandable or logical.

DR. KONDROT: How do you determine what homeopathic substances to use, or how do you determine what toxic substance is affecting them? Do you use specialized testing?

DR. COWDEN: When I first started doing this back in 2001, I was using muscle testing so I could fine-tune every step, and it was a very laborious process. It would take about two hours to do the testing to figure out what we needed to treat. It got even more frustrating when I tried to teach that to other practitioners. I found a device that I could program that would do the testing in an automated fashion. That was a ZYTO device. With this device, the patient puts their hand on an electrode; the electrode is attached to a computer, and the computer does an automated galvanic skin response test. It takes about 10 or 15 minutes and the secretary or receptionist can run the machine.

Once you have this data, the technician puts vials of water in front of the equipment. The machine, having previously stored the imprints of many, many homeopathic remedies, now transmits these frequencies — the frequencies of the substances needed by the patient — in the vials of water. They are then essentially homeopathic medicine. We use these in conjunction with the laser treatment.

DR. KONDROT: That sounds like it's something I'm going to have to investigate because I've been using the ZYTO machine to evaluate allergies and heavy metal, so it would be just a simple application to experiment with your particular method to see how effective the detoxification is.

DR. COWDEN: We find that it helps to deal with not just toxicities and autoimmunities, as I mentioned, but also with food allergies. I used to do NAET or the Nabudripad's Allergy Elimination Technique to get rid of food allergies, and I found that the laser sweep worked just as well, but you can get rid of all the food allergies in one session rather than going through 20 or 30 sessions with the NAET.

DR. KONDROT: I know that you have a great interest in Lyme disease. The Lyme organism is mimicking many medical conditions, so you feel strongly that more doctors should be focusing on it.

DR. COWDEN: I became interested in Lyme disease in 2002 when a naturopathic friend of mine brought her grandson to see me when I was hosting a conference. This boy had been an *A* student, an avid athlete, and had been exposed to the *Borrelia* microorganism and had gone straight downhill. He became an *F* student and couldn't even get out of bed or go to school.

A physician tested him and found that he had *Borrelia* antibodies in his bloodstream, started him on pharmaceutical antibiotics, and the boy got progressively worse instead of better, which is commonly the case. *Borrelia* is a spiral-shaped bacterium that is related to the one that causes syphilis, *Treponema pallidum*.

3. Lyme disease can mimic 350 or more diseases and can be transmitted many ways, not just from ticks.

Borrelia is very invasive in the body, and it's called the second great imitator. It can imitate several hundred different diseases. A website with a science library about this is www.Nutramedix.ec. One of the last articles in the science library is an article that shows more than 350 conditions that Lyme disease mimics. Those are neurological conditions and rheumotological conditions such as joint and arthritic conditions, musculoskeletal conditions, fibromyalgia, chronic fatigue, a variety of gastrointestinal conditions, and a variety of cardiovascular conditions. It's a huge problem that is unfortunately going unrecognized for the most part in the United States.

DR. KONDROT: What percent of the population do you feel is misdiagnosed?

DR. COWDEN: It's my estimate that the number of cases that are reported — and it is a reportable illness, by the way — is only about 10% of those that actually occur. The reason I say that is because the veterinarians in the United States are diagnosing Lyme disease at a rate of about ten times the rate in dogs that the medical doctors are diagnosing it in humans that live in the same household.

We're taught as allopathic physicians that Lyme disease is only transmitted by tick bites from a specific type of tick. That's probably not true. There are some reports in the literature that show the *Borrelia* and the co-infections that go with it have been transmitted by the bites of fleas, lice, and even mosquitoes, and that there is live *Borrelia* found in the saliva, so it may be transmitted by kissing.

Live *Borrelia* is found in semen and vaginal secretions, so it's probably transmitted by sexual intercourse. The live *Borrelia* is found in banked blood, so it's probably transmitted by blood transfusions. The *Borrelia* is found in breast milk and unpasteurized milk from cows and goats, so it can probably be transmitted that way as well.

There's pretty good evidence that it's transmitted from the mom, through the placenta into the fetus, so all the time the fetus is growing in the womb, it's being infected by the *Borrelia*.

The *Borrelia* is not the only culprit. In most cases when somebody gets Lyme disease, they get *Borrelia* plus at least one other co-infection microbe. In the case of this boy whom I described, it was *Borrelia* plus cytomegalovirus and maybe others that we didn't recognize.

Commonly it's *Borrelia* plus *Bartonella,* which causes cat scratch fever and a variety of other illnesses, or *Babesia,* which causes an illness like malaria with night sweats, fatigue, and neurological symptoms. It also can be some of the *Rickettsia,* the ones that cause Rocky Mountain spotted fever, *Anaplasma, Coxiella,* or *Ehrlichia.*

There are a lot of different bugs that go along with these, and collectively they cause a variety of symptoms. There are a lot of people out there with mysterious illnesses, and the doctors don't know what's going on with them. The doctors haven't thought about Lyme disease or done a test for Lyme disease because the patient doesn't have the appropriate history.

DR. KONDROT: It sounds like it's an epidemic right in front of our eyes, and we should be doing routine testing on all of our sick patients.

DR. COWDEN: Yes, I think we should. The labs that do the testing are not that good at finding the bugs, unfortunately, at least the *Borrelia* bugs.

Dr. William Harvey and Dr. Patricia Salvato in Houston, Texas, in 2000 or 2001 had 455 patients in their practice with chronic fatigue and a variety of other symptoms. Every patient had multiple symptoms. Dr. Harvey had been labeled as having Amyotrophic Lateral Sclerosis himself and had recovered from it by taking high doses of intravenous antibiotics for the *Borrelia* that he also had. He thought, "Maybe my patients have *Borrelia* that's been undiagnosed," so he tested those 455 patients.

On the first test, one third of them were positive for *Borrelia*. He wondered if the test missed any of the remaining two thirds, so he did a second test on them and found that a significant percentage were positive. Then he did a third test on the ones who were negative the second time and found some more that were positive.

Over the course of a year, almost all of those 455 patients were positive for *Borrelia*. It just shows how difficult the thing is to diagnose. I think some of those patients had to have six or eight blood tests to find it.

The bugs live inside the cells, not outside the cells, and typically the test is an antibody test to determine what's going on in the blood serum, and the bugs are not in the serum. That's one of the reasons why it's hard to diagnose.

DR. KONDROT: You advise repeated testing. I know you're a big advocate of electrodermal testing. Does that have any value in diagnosing this problem?

DR. COWDEN: Absolutely. Most of the laboratory tests in the United States are for the *Borrelia burgdorferi*. That's the most virulent form of *Borrelia,* but there are 36 species of *Borrelia* that are known to invade humans. The other ones that are highly virulent are the *Borrelia afzelii* and the *Borrelia garinii*. Those are more common in Europe, but they are also found here in the United States.

Most labs don't even look for any of those *Borrelias*. I've found on the ZYTO testing that we can actually test for 24 of them. We have the energy imprint of 24 different *Borrelia* species in our equipment, so we can find the vast majority of them with electrodermal screening, or we can at least get a clue that they might be there. If you get a clue that they might be there, you have two choices at that point. You can keep doing repeated blood testing until you find it or start the patient on a low-risk, low-expense empiric treatment program and see if they get well. If they get well, you conclude that they probably had it.

DR. KONDROT: You were explaining how accurate you felt the ZYTO electrodermal testing is for it.

DR. COWDEN: According to the research project that was done in Beijing at a large hospital, the correlation with conventional testing is 87%. That's not 100%. It shouldn't really be considered a laboratory test. It's just a guess improver, but it's pretty good. I think it's worthwhile to have the energetic (electrodermal) test done if the blood tests are negative and see what that shows. The doctor then can make a decision whether to do empiric treatment for the suspected Lyme disease.

DR. KONDROT: It seems that this condition can be so devastating and so debilitating that you're better off instituting treatment even if you're just suspicious. Many times the laboratory test is negative when, in fact, the individual still harbors the organism that may be causing many peculiar medical problems like fibromyalgia, weakness, and neurological problems, perhaps even macular degeneration and inflammation of the eye.

DR. COWDEN: Most allopathic doctors, when they diagnose Lyme disease, put the patient on two weeks of pharmaceutical antibiotics per the recommendation of the Infectious Diseases Society of America. The patients in some cases get better. In some cases they don't. At the end of two weeks, and definitely no more than four weeks, the Infectious Diseases Society of America says that the treatment's finished and that no matter what the patient's symptoms are, you shouldn't give any more treatment with pharmaceutical antibiotics.

That's a problem because what are those patients who are still ill supposed to do? They can't get their insurance to pay for anything that's outside of the guidelines of the Infectious Diseases Society of America. What we found is that the program we originally developed for the young boy whom I mentioned earlier — an herbal program — actually works both for patients who have had antibiotics already and for patients who have never had antibiotics for Lyme disease.

With an herbal program, you're talking about less risk. There's very little risk of toxicity. The only toxicity we ever see is what's called a Herxheimer reaction, which means that the bugs are dying off so rapidly that the carcasses are piling up in the tissues and making the patient feel a bit ill.

The herbal treatment is not terribly expensive either. It's something that some patients even do on their own without the guidance of a doctor. Some patients search and search to try to find a doctor who will help them with their Lyme condition and can't find one. They finally just resort to self-help.

DR. KONDROT: It's hard to believe that a simple herbal treatment can be more effective than powerful antibiotics. Part of this doesn't surprise me. On the other hand, I still have some disbelief. Are these common herbal products or a customized formula?

DR. COWDEN: There's a variety of different formulas that would have an effect against *Borrelia*, but the ones that have been studied at the University of New Haven of Connecticut by Dr. Eva Sapi and her group are Banderol which is the bark off of a Peruvian tree, in an alcohol extract, and Samento, which is the extract of the Peruvian cat's claw plant, also from the rainforest.

The two of those together have been shown by Dr. Sapi to eliminate all forms of *Borrelia*, the spirochete form which is this spiral shaped bacteria, the round body form which is a little granular form that develops very soon after exposure to antibiotics, and then the biofilm form which is probably one of the most common forms in the body. A biofilm form is like a big glob of snot with bugs growing inside of it. These bugs are capable of producing this mucopolysaccharide globus that they inhabit and that shields them from the immune system and a lot of the pharmaceutical antibiotics. The study that was done by Dr. Sapi at the University of New Haven showed that the combination of Banderol and Samento are more effective in getting rid of the biofilm by far than any pharmaceutical antibiotic that she tested.

DR. KONDROT: Do homeopathic preparations have any effect?

DR. COWDEN: Homeopathic preparations do have some effect and some benefit. Those herbals that I was just mentioning are actually all quantum-physically imprinted. They act like a homeopathic and an herbal at the same moment. That's one of the reasons why they're so effective.

For the program I developed, we did a research study in Dallas on Lyme disease. It was a program designed to determine what would help people who had failed antibiotic therapy for Lyme disease. When we did an 18-week study, we found that the patients in our integrative treatment group, who were getting a lot of different all-natural therapies, had fairly dramatic improvement whereas the patients in the control group who were being treated with allopathic pharmaceutical treatments had almost no improvement.

The study never got published. It was a pilot study, but we learned a lot from that study and continued to follow some of those patients. One of the patients was a 35-year-old man who was completely disabled and told by two doctors there was no hope for ever getting well. He had already seen 50 physicians and had taken two trips to the Mayo Clinic.

During the research protocol, he actually got pretty well over 18 weeks. In nine months' time, he was actually able to build a house with his own hands. Then he became a naturopathic doctor and is now helping other patients do the treatment for Lyme disease and so on.

Another young woman in the program

was 18 years old, was homebound, home-schooled, and ill for 15 years. She got ill when she was three years old. She walked with a walker and had recurrent anaphylactic shock reactions to foods and was in pretty bad shape. She was told that she'd never go to college and never, ever marry.

She continued the treatment program. By the ninth month, she was able to go to college and work her way through college with honors in four years. Then she got her master's degree and got married. Now she's working on a PhD degree.

We showed that there is some hope for people who do a natural treatment program even though there's no hope given to them by allopathic doctors who failed to get them well with the pharmaceutical antibiotics.

DR. KONDROT: Those cases are truly amazing. I wonder if you can give some information about these programs

DR. COWDEN: Courses about the Cowden Support Program, about Laser Detox, about EVOX, and other therapeutic and diagnostic tools used in integrative medicine can be found at www.ACIM-connect.com, (The Academy of Comprehensive Integrative Medicine). There are several membership levels in this organization, and some levels offer free courses. The Bionatus website in Ecuador, www.NutraMedix.ec, has a lot of information about the Cowden Support Program from the distributor of the NutraMedix products in Ecuador. Most of the products needed for the Cowden Support Program are produced by the NutraMedix company in Jupiter, Florida. I have no ownership in NutraMedix, but I do some consulting work for them.

Some people may have conditions for which conventional doctors have no help or hope. They may choose to contact the Academy through the email address info @ACIMConnect.com because we may know a practitioner somewhere in the world who has solutions for almost every condition.

Even though I have not had any patients of my own since 2009, I educate many healthcare practitioners, with the hope that more practitioners will become comfortable taking care of patients given no help or hope by the conventional medical system.

....

W. Lee Cowden, MD, MD(H)
Flower Mound, Texas
www.acimconnect.com

Garry F. Gordon, DO, MD, MD(H)

PAYSON, ARIZONA

Interviewed July 28, 2013

1. The F.I.G.H.T. For Your Health program, if followed faithfully, can give you vibrant health into your second century!

2. Genes may be 20% of the equation, but environment is 80% of the story.

3. As energetic beings, our thoughts and emotions radiate vibrational signals, and those signals can affect us physically.

4. Regenerative medicine goes far beyond anti-aging; it actually reverses aging.

DR. KONDROT: Dr. Gordon is a good friend of mine and a prominent national alternative doctor. For those who may not be familiar with you, tell us about your medical career and how you got interested in alternative and integrative medicine.

DR. GORDON: The good Lord gave me a very unhealthy body. I was born very sick and had almost everything going wrong, from underdeveloped testicles with very low testosterone, to no stomach acid, to metabolic problems, vision problems, fragile bones and joints, and a very weak heart. As a young boy, I suffered from repeated high fevers, which weakened my teeth. Consequently, most of my teeth needed fillings and, of course, they were mercury. The next dentist I saw said they did it all wrong. So he took the mercury out, and put in all fresh mercury. I spent that year pretty much in an unconscious state with mercury poisoning, but in those years no one knew about mercury toxicity, so they called it narcolepsy.

I have had bilateral carpal tunnel syndrome, with my hands so painful and numb all night that I could not sleep. I've had back pain so bad, that I needed a hook on the wall just to get off the toilet. I was born with a heart defect, so I was never able to participate in sports, ride a bike, or swim even one lap.

Now at age 79, I research and practice regenerative medicine, and I enjoy the best health of my lifetime. Those health challenges led me to a lifetime pursuit of answers about how to get healthy. In the 55 years I've been a licensed physician, I have attended meetings on every health topic in many countries around the world.

The result is that I am motivated and eager to tell everyone that, no matter what seems to be wrong with you, there are alternative doctors who have real answers! Of course, all of us are hoping to find a magic bullet. I haven't necessarily found one, but armed with 50-plus years of research and experience, I have developed a basic program that has worked wonders in the lives of thousands of my patients, and in my life too!

There is no one magic bullet that's going to let you live to your maximum intended useful life span, which many today think that is only somewhere between 75 and 85 years, but I know that we can live full and healthy lives for much longer than that! It is possible to live and thrive upwards of 90 to 120 years! There is emerging science in the field of regenerative medicine that is helping us to grow ever healthier and live far longer than we dreamed possible. But you're not going to reach your maximum intended life span, enjoying optimal health, without doing prevention and maintenance.

I have developed an owner's manual for the human body. It's now my job to share that approach with as many people as possible. I've done the legwork, and found some really useful answers, and I want to help others reap the benefits that I have, without the slow and expensive learning process.

DR. KONDROT: One thing I really admire about you, Dr. Gordon, is that you walk the talk. I am shocked when you reveal that you're 79 years of age. When I see you at meetings, you have so much energy. Tell me a little bit about what you do and your approach to disease.

DR. GORDON: My father was what is traditionally known as a ten-fingered osteopath, meaning that his treatment and healing were done primarily through manipulation of the patient's body. He was very gifted in healing patients. His practice was in Madison, Wisconsin, where he treated people rejected from the Mayo clinic, including a young man with multiple sclerosis. No one had been able to help him. We helped this young man fully recover, without any drugs but primarily with a lifestyle program.

So by the time I decided to become a physician, I knew that mainstream medicine did not have all the answers. My practice today is very eclectic. I take patients off most drugs very rapidly. I don't like the side effects of drugs, and I don't believe that drugs are the best answer. What's different about my practice is that I have sought the best answers for health and healing from around the world; I have spent millions of dollars over the past 55 years, as a researcher, a practicing physician, and expert consultant, having taught and lectured at conferences on every continent. All of this knowledge and experience I now freely share through my free on-line FACT MEMBERSHIP program which is open to health practitioners.

I have also become what I call a "second opinion" consultant for patients who have been told that nothing else can be done for them. I always find something that the other doctors or their mainstream medical team haven't considered. It doesn't matter if they've been to Hopkins or Mayo and have seen the "best," I've always found something that got left out. I come along like Sherlock Holmes and solve the mystery. But there is never just one culprit; the contributors to impaired health are usually multifactorial.

It's not just that you need vitamin C, or that you need to get off gluten, or be put on testosterone, or just need to exercise. We are all very toxic since we have poisoned our planet, and so have poisoned ourselves. If we're going to reach that magical 90 to 120 years of age still functioning and feeling good, we need to expend the effort to detoxify and replenish on a daily basis for life.

1. The F.I.G.H.T. For Your Health program, if followed faithfully, can give you vibrant health into your second century!

This is why I've developed my F.I.G.H.T. FOR YOUR HEALTH program as a safe and simple way to deal with the multi-factorial nature of illness and disease. F.I.G.H.T. is an acronym, which stands for Food & Focus, Infection, Genetics, Heavy Metals, Hormones, and Toxins. By addressing each of these simultaneously, we are able to correct underlying problems and allow our bodies to heal naturally.

2. Genes may be 20% of the equation, but environment is 80% of the story.

While striving to solve the problems of my own ill health, I had to look at my genetics. I've had a personal DNA profile done, and it shows that I have various genes that predispose me to certain conditions. For instance, I have genes indicating a high risk of developing cardiovascular disease, metabolic syndrome, of having an impaired pancreatic-insulin function, vitamin D insufficiency, and an increased risk for pro-carcinogenic activation. I have issues with two-thirds of the genes tested. While we know that many illnesses have a genetic component, we also know today that possessing a particular gene does not mean that you need to develop any particular condition including breast cancer. Genes may be 20% of the equation, but environment is 80% of the story. It is our environment that determines whether that gene expresses itself or not. That is great news because we have some control over our environment.

It is scary to be told that you have cancer and are offered a poisonous drug, a drug that is itself a known carcinogen, that kills your immune system, and makes your hair fall out. How is it they think another poison is going to cure you? Otto Warburg, a top scientist in Europe, got the Nobel Prize in 1931 for explaining cancer's origin, and conventional options are not the answer. Researchers are wisely revisiting Warburg's hypothesis that claims that cancer is a metabolic disease, not a genetic one, and it is curable! Early diagnosis is available today at caprofile. net. The ONCOblot test is a blood test that is apparently 100% accurate, so no one needs to undergo repeated cat scans to know when they are free of cancer.

The cost of genetic testing is coming down so fast that most of us very soon will be able to afford it. With these tests, you may find that regardless of what doctor you've seen, they have missed a key piece of the puzzle. It could be toxic overload, infections, or something like defective methylation.

The Mount Sinai School of Medicine toxin screen, where for $4,900 and 20 tubes of blood, will measure your body burden of more than 220 toxins. Even if your family lived to 90 or 100 without Alzheimer's or cancer, you will not be as healthy as they were because these toxins have caused some of your genes to operate inefficiently in the important area of detoxification. For example, Biphenyl A interferes with DNA methylation, which controls DNA expression.

All of us have some of these issues, and toxins can induce epigenetic changes that set the stage for health problems our parents did not have. What is so exciting is that my detox and chelation protocols have shown they can help protect against, and even reverse, many of these changes.

I am known as the "Father of Chelation" because I helped write the protocol to avoid heart surgery like bypass operations by using chelation therapy to remove the lead we are all born with. Approximately 10 million people have safely canceled bypass surgery and even amputations of gangrenous feet through chelation therapy. I've improved chelation to the point now that we can all do it safely orally, every day of our lives. I really like intravenous chelation, too, as that is a great way to start a serious detox program, but I don't have to do IV chelation to keep patients with serious heart blockages alive. I cancel bypass procedures on all of my patients, and none of my patients get a stent. None of my patients are on statins. Most doctors blame cholesterol for everything, which is so misguided, since cholesterol is essential for health. Some studies indicate that a higher level of cholesterol is actually associated with longer life. The fact is that cholesterol has little to do with fatal heart attacks; blood clots are the problem.

The oral chelation that I designed, that I call Beyond Chelation Improved, or BC-I, is an all-natural nutritional supplement package of nine pills that works to prevent excessive blood clotting, as aspirin is supposed to do, but BC-I is safer and without the harmful side effects associated with long-term aspirin therapy or other blood thinning drugs like Coumadin and Plavix. Aspirin is really too weak for meaningful blood thinning, and Coumadin is too dangerous.

The success of this program is due to many things including helping lower blood clotting tendencies as well as the body's burden of lead and mercury. All of us have 1,000 to 2,000 times more lead in our bones at birth than those born before the industrial age, and it begins to accumulate in utero. BC-I does much more than chelation; it also has resveratrol, that has been shown to reduce inflammation, reduce LDL cholesterol and prevent blood clots, and vitamin K2, which works to lower the levels of calcium in the arteries, helping to keep arterial walls soft while keeping our bones strong. I believe everyone today *needs* vitamin K2, at least 90 mcgs a day, if they hope to maintain strong bones and avoid the hardened, calcified arteries that we see in nearly everyone by age 80.

As we age, our tissues calcify as we lose calcium from our bones. In later years, our aorta has turned to stone! We have on average 140 times more calcium in the aorta than was present at age ten; while at the same time, our bones are getting weaker and losing calcium. Vitamin K2 is one of the keys to preventing this.

So BC-I is a total regimen of nine capsules that includes three very powerful vitamin and mineral tablets with resveratrol, three Essential Daily Defense capsules, which combine EDTA, garlic, and sulfated mucopolysaccharides from carrageenan, one Omega-3 fish oil capsule, one 1300 mg capsule of primrose oil, and one capsule containing gingko biloba and phosphatidylserine.

I recommend chelation to everyone as the way to help your body get rid of lead! Comparing my BC-I formula to recent studies saying that taking a multiple vitamin is a waste of money is like comparing a little red wagon to a Lear jet. Drug companies delight in confusing the public that nutritional supplements are wasting money. The *JAMA* reported years ago that drugs prescribed by your physician are the fourth leading cause of death in America. I believe today they would be recognized as the leading cause of death if proper studies were done.

I've outlined my chelation protocols in detail, in a chapter entitled "The Natural, Effective Alternative to Bypass Surgery," in Suzanne Somer's book *Bombshell*. It doesn't matter if your doctor says, "You're a heart attack waiting to happen." I consider them all badly misinformed.

Just as I do not believe in standard heart treatment today, I also do not agree with most doctors today on cancer treatment. I don't have any of my patients do the chemo-radiation-surgery approach because Thomas Seyfried, a top researcher at Boston University, documents that cancer is a metabolic disease. A book by Laura Bond, *Mum's Not Having Chemo: Cutting-Edge Therapies, Real-Life Stories, a Road-Map to Healing from Cancer*, will help you understand how useless I consider chemo and radiation. This book explains that there are far better answers than those available through conventional medicine.

Mainstream cancer care offers 2 to 3% of their metastatic patients a five-year survival; whereas my colleagues around the world have proven that 30 to 70% can have a five-year survival. We are lucky to have alternative doctors worldwide whose results are getting better by the day, as long as we *avoid* mainstream cancer care.

When I do a second opinion consultation on patients from around the world today, I seldom agree with the medical opinion given them by their primary physician, because my experience and training and treatment successes have allowed me to look at things very differently.

DR. KONDROT: Dr. Gordon, I think that your F.I.G.H.T. program is so important. I wonder if you could go over that in detail because I think it epitomizes your practice and your approach.

DR. GORDON: Dr. Tsuneo Kobayashi, who's a molecular biologist, MD, PhD, oncologist and pathologist in Japan, was funded by the Sun Moon Church to follow 10,000 patients for ten years, and, by placing them on his holistic health program and having annual screenings, he proved that no one has to die of cancer. I guess you could say that my F.I.G.H.T. program is the Americanized version of the Kobayashi program. F.I.G.H.T. is an acronym that helps to remind us of the multifactorial nature of illness, and what areas of change or care we need to focus upon on a daily basis.

So "F" stands for Food; technically there would be two Fs, one for food and the second one for focus. Our food supply no longer gives us the nutrients that we need. Because of this, I believe we all need to take food supplements. Logically we should all be avoiding high fructose corn syrup (HFCS), aspartame, fluoride, genetically modified organisms (GMO), irradiated, over-processed and fast foods. Leaky gut syndrome and GERD (reflux disease) is almost unavoidable with the GMO, HFCS, soy, and corn in everyone's diet, providing a pesticide effect in our intestines and altering our flora. We should eat organic whole foods whenever possible.

I realize everyone's dietary needs are not the same, however, and finding the most beneficial combination of foods and supplements can be complex. It is estimated that more than 50% of people have some kind of food allergy or sensitivity that could be causing or contributing to illness, and it is believed that nearly 40% of us have some adverse reactions to either dairy or gluten or both.

Good news is there are several ways to determine food sensitivities. One of the best methods is through an elimination or challenge diet, where you avoid certain foods and food additives. After at least two weeks on the diet, single food items are added back in while keeping a careful diary and any adverse symptoms experienced. I also recommend the book, *The Blood Sugar Solution,* by Dr. Mark Hyman. It has 14 self-assessment health quizzes, which can help determine where your specific health challenges lie. There are quizzes on adrenal fatigue, energy, metabolism, inflammation, vitamin D, magnesium, oxidative stress, thyroid function, toxicity, and a comprehensive "diabesity" quiz. You will be more motivated to develop and stick to your own plan once you understand your challenges.

Clearly some of us do better with an all plant-based diet, and others seem to do better with other diets. Determining the ideal mix of foods for you is not a simple process. I recommend a good quality probiotic, like Kyolic's Kyo-Dophilus 9 formula, and for fiber my patients take Longevity Plus Beyond Fiber with stabilized rice bran and inulin.

3. As energetic beings, our thoughts and emotions radiate vibrational signals, and those signals can affect us physically.

The focus aspect of F.I.G.H.T. teaches that our mental and emotional state is extremely important in being healthy. It goes far beyond traditional positive thinking and into the realm of quantum mechanics, where we understand that the electromagnetic frequencies generated by our thoughts have powerful effects on our physiology. What that means is that, as energetic beings, our thoughts and emotions radiate vibrational signals, and those signals can affect us physically, and they can affect people and things around us. We need to develop and maintain a positive mindset and learn ways to reduce our stress levels.

In Bruce Lipton's books, *The Biology of Belief and Spontaneous Evolution*, he suggests that our emotions impact us genetically: that signals originating from our thoughts can actually control our DNA. And in the book *Soul Medicine*, by Norman Shealy, MD, Ph.D., he talks about the power of spiritual connections, and how our intentions, through faith and prayer, have the ability to alter our body's energy fields. Whether it is through traditional prayer, or meditation, or daily positive affirmations, striving to cultivate an attitude of love and gratitude is absolutely essential in helping to prevent sickness.

The "I" in F.I.G.H.T. is for the Infections that everybody carries, that are often inadequately diagnosed. The list of infections is a long one, with AIDS, CMV (Cytomegalovirus), H1N1, MRSA, SARS, C-diff (*Clostridium difficile*), as just a few of the thousands of pathogens encountered today. This is really just the tip of the iceberg because if you do not have candida, cytomegalovirus, Coxsackie virus, chlamydia, or Lyme disease, odds are you will acquire something else like a parasite. These undiagnosed infections are contributing to the most chronic and widespread disease including cancer. CMV is reported to be linked to heart disease and hypertension. Chlamydia has also been linked to heart disease, arterial plaque, asthma, Alzheimer's disease, and a shortened lifespan.

Coupled with our devitalized food and toxic environment, our polluted bodies lose the ability to fight off these pathogenic invaders. Over time, this constant barrage wears down our immune system, allowing the infections to dig in even deeper, leading to chronic inflammation that leads to degenerative diseases.

Remedies for infection that I like to recommend include regular use of Ozone in any form. Also I never go without supplements like Advanced Cellular Silver 200 (ACS 200) and my Bio En'R-G'y C formula. When used properly, ACS 200 can help the body eliminate all known pathogens, including MRSA, *Candida albicans*, and even *Borrelia burgdorferi* that causes Lyme disease. At proper levels, higher than the RDA says you need, vitamin C has antihistamine,

antitoxin, antibiotic, and antiviral properties. Since most people are vitamin D deficient, I recommend a daily dose of D3 at 3,000-5,000 units per day as the ideal adult target dose. Vitamin D supports the immune system and helps reduce the incidence of cancer, diabetes, arthritis, and hypertension.

Genetics is what the "G" in F.I.G.H.T. stands for. Because of our toxic load, we all have genes that have changed; this is called epigenetic change. We don't methylate well, and that's a big word, but it really means that our bodies are not detoxing as well as they should. Biphenyl A, or BPA, that's used to make water bottles, plastic wraps, resin coatings in food and beverage cans, is just one of the many toxins we are exposed to on a daily basis. BPA is an endocrine disruptor, which can mimic the body's own hormones and cause many negative health effects.

In one study, a group of pregnant Agouti mice were exposed to BPA. A high percentage of their offspring were born yellow and predisposed to obesity and diabetes and heart disease. Sounds like what is happening to our children and us today doesn't it? When these sickly, yellow Agouti mice were given methyl-rich supplements like folic acid and vitamin B12, they gave birth to offspring that were lean, brown, and healthy. These nutrients were able to reverse the epigenetic defects! Most people have been exposed to BPA. Medical research reveals that 95% of patients have BPA in their urine, and this breakthrough research may help explain today's epidemic of obesity, diabetes, and cancer.

Just because you have certain genes doesn't mean you will become diseased. Angelina Jolie had her breasts removed, as a "preventative" measure, because she has the gene for breast cancer called BRCA. She will probably have her ovaries removed as well. Sadly, that decision was based on very bad information she's received from mainstream medicine. She didn't have breast cancer, and doesn't have ovarian cancer. I see these preventative surgeries as an unnecessary mutilation, because even with breasts and ovaries removed she will still carry the risk unless she goes on a total life-extending program that I am describing here.

Continuing with the F.I.G.H.T. acronym, The "H" represents two different categories, one for heavy metals, and the other for Hormones. My chelation protocol was initially developed through my extensive studies on heavy metal toxicity, and I opened the major laboratories in Asia, Europe, and the U.S. to measure lead, mercury, cadmium, and selenium and zinc levels in human blood, urine, and hair. Heavy metals are found in nearly everyone on the planet. Mercury toxicity from vaccines and amalgam fillings are linked to autism and other neurological disorders, and heavy metal exposure is linked to Alzheimer's, which is predicted to affect one in two people by age 80.

Heavy metal exposure suppresses the immune system. Most don't realize how pervasive this really is. Lead is commonly found in cosmetics, toothpaste, and water. We know about mercury in fish and dental amalgams, but it also exists in many adhesives, and in things like Preparation H, psoriasis ointments, contact lens solution, vaginal lubricants, and tattoo dyes. Arsenic, which may be associated with Type II diabetes, is commonly found in chicken meat due to additives in the chicken feed. Aluminum is present in many antiperspirants and has been associated with Alzheimer's disease and ALS. Cadmium is found in cigarette smoke, processed meats, and instant coffee.

High levels of lead have been associated with aggressive behavior in children and high blood pressure in adults. Men with high levels of lead in their bones are six times more likely to die from cardiovascular disease. Stenting and bypass surgery are of limited value, as blockages exist throughout the body, not just in the vicinity of the heart, which is why chelation therapy is needed. I'm sure Dr. Kondrot is familiar with the 2004 study that associates lead exposure with age-related cataracts in men. This study provides proof that bone lead levels are adversely affecting the health of the brain, as the eye is an extension of the brain. Even more frightening is that there is a synergistic effect when both lead and mercury are present together which results in them being *100 times* more toxic than when either exists alone. And fluoride, added to toothpaste and in most all municipal drinking water, increases heavy metal accumulation in the bones and tissues.

There are tests today that can identify who is likely to die of a heart attack and who is not. We don't need the hospital or an angiogram. All we need is a multifunction cardiogram based on www.Premier-Heart.com. This simple computerized EKG tells you in five minutes whether or not you have a serious obstruction in one of your arteries. If you know about it, you'll never go off your oral chelation program and, when needed, add other natural things that prevent blood clots like lumbrokinase and serrapeptase enzymes.

"H" is for hormones too, and hormonal problems are epidemic today. Men have erectile dysfunction and low testosterone or low "T," and women are suffering and being cheated out of a full life because they've been told that if they take estrogen, then they're going to get breast cancer or have a heart attack. It's all nonsense.

We don't have to succumb to the effects of hormonal imbalance, due to the natural aging process and the adverse effects of toxins on our hormones. We have an amazing natural remedy made from an herb called *Pueraria mirifica* found in the mountainous regions of Thailand that is changing the life of every woman who's lucky enough to hear about it.

This miraculous plant contains a unique substance known as miroestrol, which is similar in structure and function to a type of estrogen called estriol. Clinical trials have shown no links between estriol and cancer. The herb produces favorable effects throughout the entire body. It is an adaptogen, acting to balance or moderate estrogenic effects. While hormone replacement therapy has been disparaged due to its links to cancers, the same is not true of miroestrol, which is why the native Thai peoples use this herb as a food and medicine and have the lowest cancer rates on the planet.

What is also amazing about the estrogenic effects of miroestrol in *Pueraria mirifica* is that it can reverse aging! It does this by increasing "telomerase" activity, lengthening our telomeres. Telomeres have been described as protective end caps on the ends of our chromosomes, and their length determines how fast we are aging.

Another exciting new therapy in the regenerative medicine realm is a telomerase-activating supplement called TA-65. This product is derived from the *Astragalus* herb, which is used a lot in traditional Chinese medicine for its beneficial effect on the immune system.

Pueraria mirifica has been studied for over 20 years and is now standardized and FDA approved as a nutritional supplement. It is also available in the United States in a formulation called HRT Plus – Herbal Remedy from Thailand. Dr. Christiane Northrup, who wrote a book called *Women's Bodies, Women's Wisdom,* is teaching women that this formulation alone has restored the elasticity of the vaginal tract for women who had suffered painful intercourse. We also have formulated it into a gel for topical vaginal application, which works wonders to moisturize and rejuvenate those areas, enhancing the pleasure of sex.

Another beneficial hormonal adaptogen for both men and women is the Peruvian root *Lepidium meyenii*, commonly known as maca. Maca root contains two groups of novel compounds, which are believed to have mood- and sex-enhancing powers. Men and women with low libido feel a boost in sexual desire, and men with erectile problems notice marked improvement in sexual function. *Pueraria mirifica* and Maca are both recommended as part of my F.I.G.H.T. For Your Health program.

Lastly, there is the letter "T" for Toxins. This is the elephant in the living room. It is the big problem, and one that encompasses all the categories in F.I.G.H.T. Not long ago, the Environmental Working Group released the video *10 Americans,* which looks at the impact of environmental toxicity on ten of America's children. In the study, 287 chemicals were found in the ten randomly chosen participants with an average of 200 chemicals in each child: 134 of the chemicals have been shown to cause cancer; 151 are known to cause birth defects; 186 have been associated with infertility; 154 cause hormone disruption; 130 are toxic to the immune system; 158 are known neurotoxins that have profound effects on develop-

ing children. More surprisingly, 212 of the chemicals and pesticides had been banned in the United States over 30 years before the study was conducted.

We've poisoned our Mother Earth. We've done it at a time when we are really facing a secondary challenge of magnetic changes, where the North Pole may someday become South Pole. That's why we experience some increasingly strange weather patterns and other intense geological events. Climate change and magnetic pole changes have occurred hundreds of times over the last few million years; the poles typically reverse every 200,000 or 300,000 years, and we are overdue for one currently. Why this is important as far as our health is concerned is that the earth's electro-magnetic field affects how our bodies function. Every living organism on the planet has evolved under its influence. As the planet has been preparing for a reversal, its electro-magnetic field has been weakening, decreasing by as much as 10% over the past 150 years. And as it has weakened, it has affected us physiologically. The proper electromagnetic frequencies are necessary for our body's energy production, but also necessary in modulating our circadian rhythms, for healthy immune function, and they also affect how we perceive pain.

Here is where the exciting field of energy medicine, particularly pulsed electromagnetic frequency therapy or PEMF, comes in! PEMF has literally given me a brand new spine and back, and this therapy, coupled with my enhanced

Zeogold with Hydrogen supplement, has given me a stronger and normally functioning heart; gone are my atrial fibrillation symptoms.

PEMF is like an advanced form of exercise; I call it M.I.C.E., which is short for "magnetically induced cellular exercise," because it works on a cellular level and produces the same effect and benefit as hard physical exercise, but without the stress and strain on our muscles and bones. This is so important because we have learned that exercise is necessary for cellular detoxification and renewal. PEMF provides the energy for "electroporation" to occur, whereby small pores in the cells outer membrane are opened to allow toxins to be expelled, and vital nutrients and oxygen to be taken in! PEMF therapy also stimulates stem cell production, and is a key therapy in regenerative medicine.

I also strongly recommend my Power Drink for detoxification and nutrient supplementation; it's like the F.I.G.H.T. program in a glass! The Power Drink contains my Beyond Fiber, Best of Organic Greens, Bio En'R-G'y C, Maca, and Zeogold Enhanced supplements and is a very convenient way to address all the aspects together.

4. Regenerative medicine goes far beyond anti-aging; it actually reverses aging.

As Dr. Kondrot was kind enough to say, at age 79, I don't look that age, and I certainly don't feel it, because I do walk the talk. I am living proof of the power of regenerative medicine. That's a stronger word than anti-aging, because today we are no longer just slowing down the aging process; we are discovering ways to reverse it. When you're born sick, you have to do more than just stop your aging because who wants to live to 100 if you're just barely surviving? I had to find a way to make each of my issues go away, and now my hands aren't numb, my back isn't killing me, and my heart is allowing me to ride my bicycle uphill.

To feel as good as I do at 79, I take a lot of supplements. But I know what to take. It's my job to help people know what they need to do, so they don't have to waste money taking a lot of one thing, while missing all the other things that are necessary. I help people learn to use a magnet to exercise part of their body, so that part of their body will bring in stem cells to regenerate their bad back. You don't need a back operation, knee or hip replacement when we teach other methods.

If I could change the laws in this country, I would change it so that patients would have the right to get ozone; high-dose vitamin C; Salvestrols, which are like the body's police force to manage threats; and some of my other favorite therapies. I love educating my patients and other doctors and sharing all the research and knowledge that has helped me to regenerate my body and reclaim my health. Regenerative medicine is producing miraculous treatments, such as the research from Dr. Stephen Badylak at the McGowan Center for Regenerative Medicine at the University of Pittsburgh. He created a miraculous substance made from pig bladder called extracellular matrix or "pixie dust." This powder can actually cause human cells and tissues to regrow! One of his patients, a military war veteran who had his quadriceps muscles blown away by an explosive device, was actually able to regenerate and grow back these muscles. Recently reported in the news, is how gene-therapy completely cured an eight-year-old girl from terminal late-stage cancer! Known as T-cell gene therapy, doctors use this treatment to transform the patients' blood cells into "soldiers" that seek and destroy their cancer.

Over 3,000 clinicians from around the world communicate with each other on a daily basis through the FACT (Forum on Anti-aging and Chelation Therapies and share their experiences and successes in alternative therapies on my website. It is totally free.

We have real answers, successful natural treatments, and I've endeavored to provide these answers to everyone. I have power point webinars and presentations available on my website, www.gordonresearch.com, that reveal the latest studies and documentation so that you know your options.

You don't have to wonder, "Do I have infections?" Yes, you do. You don't have to wonder, "Do I have toxins?" Absolutely, you do. Is there any miracle program?

No. There's not a miracle program, but I have a program where I can change the water that you drink into a powerful anti-oxidative elixir, just by having you add zeolite and hydrogen to it, so that the water will work like vitamin C and vitamin E.

It has been proven already that basic things like diet, detoxing, supplementation, lowering stress, and improving your thought processes will keep your disease genes from expressing. You must follow the program faithfully for life. That means you're going to have to eat the right foods and exercise. If you want to live and still feel good at 90 or 120, my F.I.G.H.T. program will help you attain that goal.

I am happy to work with my patients to personalize their F.I.G.H.T. program, depending upon their test results.

Anyone interested in developing his or her own F.I.G.H.T. For Your Health program can request one by emailing or phoning me. My consult typically covers one-hour discussion of history and diagnostics, and I provide you with both a written and recorded copy of the phone consultation along with suggested protocols. Because I am passionate about educating others, if your primary physician is on the call, I will typically reduce my consult fee by 50%.

I can't keep you alive, keep you from having a heart attack or stroke, or keep you cancer-free without testing. You are more inclined to stay on your program if you know your risk factors. Yes, it takes

some effort, but isn't living and enjoying
a long and full life worth it?

....

Dr. Garry F. Gordon, md, do, md(h)
Gordon Research Institute
600 North Beeline Hwy
Payson, AZ 85541
(928)472-4263
info@gordonresearch.com
www.gordonresearch.com

Edward Kondrot, MD, MD(H), CCH, DHt

DADE CITY, FLORIDA

My Story

1. **There is a ten second test to determine if you are deficient in this key mineral for eye health.**

2. **Blue light at night is contributing to blindness!**

3. **What treatment that reversed Sam Snead's vision loss can help you?**

I am honored to be able to assemble the stories, as the result of my interviews, of the top alternative doctors in the United States. I count myself among them and am proud of my journey as well as that of my colleagues. This is not to say that it is easy to shift gears in mid-career and receive more training to learn a whole lot of innovative and effective techniques. But, our patients deserve us to be the scientists they believe we are. My story parallels that of many of the doctors included in this book. I hope readers will take heart and hope from reading this narrative.

I'm a board-certified ophthalmologist, and I have practiced traditional ophthalmology and surgery for 20 years. When homeopathy cured me of my severe case of asthma, I began investigating alternative treatments. Since that time, I've been integrating alternative therapies into my practice since 1990. I'm the only eye doctor in the world to be certified in ophthalmology and homeopathy. I'm the author of three bestselling books, and I'm also the host of *Healthy Vision Talk Radio*, which has been in existence for over 15 years. I have a medical license in four states, and I'm also the President of the

Arizona Homeopathic and Integrative Medical Association.

Have you been told nothing can be done to improve your vision? Have you been advised to learn to live with poor vision or that you need to give up your driver's license? We see many patients who want to tune up their vision so they can keep their wheels because one of the biggest fears seniors have is not passing that vision test to get their driver's license. The older years offer an opportunity to enjoy life with activities and grandchildren, and you certainly need good sight.

I want to be your personal coach to help your vision loss. I want to improve your eyesight, and I want you to improve the quality of your life. The Kondrot Program can improve your vision. Eighty-five percent of patients who attend The Kondrot Program boot camp will have an improvement of their vision. The program is not for everyone. It's only for those who are very serious in investing in saving their eyesight.

Unfortunately, there are problems with our healthcare system that make it difficult for people to learn about and choose some of the therapies that might save their sight. Big pharma is not our friend. They are bombarding us with toxic petrochemical pharmaceutical agents that, in many cases, cause more harm than benefit. Insurance companies dictate which treatments are approved and which are not approved. I do not always agree with their recommendations. For example, I'm a firm believer that injec-tions in the eye and surgery should be the last resort for people with eye disease. In conventional medicine, they're a first resort, often with bad consequences.

Let's begin with an outline of the program I have designed to help people keep their sight. You will notice that many of the techniques can be incorpo-rated into your life and do not need any special equipment.

FIRST IS DIET. Seventy percent of your diet should be organic, raw, or living food. Why organic? Two studies may convince you. The spinach study looked at the nutritional value of spinach in the 1940s compared to 2012. In the 1940s, the average serving of spinach had 158 milligrams of iron. In 2012, only 2.2 milligrams of iron were detected. That is really shocking and reflects our modern farming methods, petrochemicals, fer-tilizers, and pesticides, and our soil declining in its mineral value. As a result, our fruits and vegetables are declining in their nutritional value. Another study found that there were five to tenfold more nutritional elements in organic food and, interestingly, five to tenfold less toxic metal. These are two reasons to eat organic food.

Why raw or living food? Raw fruits and vegetables have much greater nutrition, because heat destroys their delicate protein structures. There's loss of amino acids and digestive enzymes. Eating raw foods is one of the best ways to shift your body chemistry to be more alkaline. We need to be in an alkaline state to support all the enzymatic reactions and chemistry in our body. Acid environments promote disease. The digestive process works better when you're alkaline. If you think raw food is not tasty, be sure to read Sal Montezinos' book, *The Raw Alkaline Cuisine.* He's an amazing chef who makes raw, living food exciting.

Non-organic food may be made of genetically modified organisms which are harmful to health. An excellent reference on this is *Seeds of Deception* written by Jeffrey Smith. A study published in the *Lancet,* England's prestigious medical journal, conclusively showed that rats fed genetically modified potatoes had a much higher incidence of developing neurological problems, cancer, failure to thrive, allergies, etc.

In Europe, most of the countries have banned GMO (genetically modified organisms) food. Mexico has banned genetically modified corn. Here in the United States, 90% of our corn is genetically modified. Eighty percent of soy products are GMO. A high percentage of canola and rapeseed oil is. By eating organic food, you are reducing the chance of consuming genetically modified food.

I trained with a doctor, Patricia Kane, who's a nutritionist in Philadelphia. One of the things that she advises all of her patients who have neurological and eye problems to do is to stop eating corn because so much of it is genetically modified.

We also need to avoid high-fructose corn syrup for several reasons. Most high-fructose corn syrup contains genetically modified corn. Second, in the manufacturing process of high-fructose corn syrup, there's an accumulation of mercury. Some alternative doctors feel there's more mercury in high-fructose corn syrup than in a tuna. High fructose corn sugar is truly not a natural sugar. It is not metabolized like glucose or sugar. It puts a greater stress on the pancreas and leads to obesity and diabetes.

I believe fish oils are contributing to your blindness. That is rather a bold statement to make. Professor Peskin researched this in great detail, and all of his work has been confirmed and supported by Dr. Robert Rowen, who is the editor of *Second Opinion* magazine. It's an excellent newsletter, and I would highly encourage you to subscribe to it. Why avoid fish oils? They're longer chain fatty acids, and they're not absorbed by the cell as readily as plant-based omegas. I'm not saying that omega oils are bad for you. I'm saying that fish-based omega oils are.

Fish oils also become rancid at room temperature, and rancid oils are toxic to the body. Fish oils do contain mercury. Some manufactures say all the mercury is removed, but I know how difficult it is to remove mercury from a human body, so I don't believe these are mercury free. I encourage you to shift to plant-based omega oils.

1. There is a 10-second test to determine if you are deficient in this key mineral for eye health.

Zinc deficiency is very common. I have found that 80% of my patients are deficient in zinc even if they're taking a zinc supplement. One reason for the deficiency may be that they're taking the wrong kind of zinc, zinc oxide that is poorly absorbed in the body. Chelated zinc is preferable. Zinc is responsible for most enzymatic reactions, and it's essential for good eye health. Several studies have been done that show that zinc deficiency leads to macular degeneration. If you wonder whether you are deficient in zinc, it is easy to find out through a very simple test you can do at home. It's the zinc tally taste test and you can order it online.

THE SECOND ITEM IN MY PROGRAM IS PROPER HYDRATION. Most of us are severely dehydrated. Dr. Batmanghelidj wrote a book called *Your Body's Many Cries for Water.* He feels that dehydration is the number one cause of chronic disease. Simply by rehydrating yourself, you can eliminate a lot of chronic problems. Hydration is necessary to remove toxins from your body. As a result of your body's metabolic processes, toxins accumulate, and they have to be cleared through proper hydration. Our general rule of thumb is that you should consume one half of your body weight in ounces of water. If you weigh 160 pounds, you should be drinking 80 ounces of water a day as a minimum.

We know the dangers of public water, including the pharmaceuticals found in it, as well as antibiotics, hormonal substances, and toxic metals. We now know the dangers of plastic bottles. The chemicals from the plastics leech into the water, so water in plastic bottles is not a good option. One good alternative is to treat your water through reverse osmosis to completely remove toxins and heavy metals. It produces almost pure distilled water. I recommend you look at investing in this in order to have a good source of water to help you regain your health and your vision.

THE THIRD IMPORTANT STEP to take is to balance your autonomic nervous system. In a state of arousal from stress certain physiological processes occur. Your pupils dilate. Your heart races; you breathe faster. Your body will not heal in this state since its resources are allocated to managing the perceive threat. Nor will it digest well. The body is fighting for its life. We need to learn to reduce stress in order to get out of this state.

Unfortunately, many times interacting with conventional medicine can induce a sympathetic state. The eye doctor tells you that if you don't have surgery or take eye drops you're going to go blind. The medical doctor tells you that if you don't have heart surgery, you're going to die. They actually put you in this fight or flight state.

One of the things we do at the Florida Wellness Center is to create an extremely relaxing environment to help you reduce your stress. That alone can contribute to your healing. How do you reduce stress? Physical exercise is good for reducing stress. Meditation, prayer, and positive affirmations are good. Some of our therapies are stress-reducing in themselves. I should probably add that we have a beautiful hot tub. Taking a nice soak at the end of the day can help your body relax and reduce stress.

THE FOURTH STEP IS WHOLE BODY EXERCISE. One of my favorite exercises for older people is the trampoline or rebounder. That is a good way to exercise at home. There have been studies showing that using a trampoline or rebounder can improve circulation to the eye. There's a technique called Exercise with Oxygen (EWO) where you exercise on a trampoline as you breathe a high flow rate of oxygen. Some alternative doctors feel that this is just as good as being in a hyperbaric chamber. This is one way of increasing oxygenation to your brain and your eye, and it has helped many patients who have eye problems like macular degeneration and glaucoma.

Dance can lower your eye pressure. I had a patient who was a professor of African dance at UCLA. He had uncontrolled glaucoma. His traditional Western eye doctors were not able to lower the pressure. I suggested he dance, and he did. He danced for 20 minutes. Believe it or not, his pressure was lowered 5 millimeters of mercury. I said, "You have to dance more."

FIFTH IS SLEEP AND LIGHT THERAPY. There is an environment which we call Light at Night (LAN), which turns out to be very harmful. I spoke with Professor Abraham Haim on *Healthy Vision Talk Radio* about the subject of LAN. You can go to the website www.HealingThe-Eye.com to listen to this interview. It is under Resources. Professor Haim looked at regions on the planet that were lit at night. Certain areas have excessive light at night, and other areas are dark. Then he studied the incidence of certain diseases that he felt were related to the circadian rhythm, meaning the innate way that all organisms respond to light and dark. He found that the incidence of breast cancer, prostate cancer, macular degeneration, heart disease and diabetes were significantly higher in areas that have light at night.

You might think that it is logical that there is a greater incidence of disease in major cities. There's stress, pollution, crowding, etc. As a control, he looked at lung cancer rates. You would think lung cancer would be statistically higher in these areas, but it was not.

He then injected breast cancer cells in a group of rats. One group was subjected to an environment of a normal diurnal change, light during the day and dark at night. The second group, he put in an environment with light at night. Not surprisingly, the group that had light at night had something like a 400% greater growth rate of the cancer. He duplicated this study looking at diabetes and heart disease. He did the same thing with prostate cancer cells and confirmed that light at night increases the growth of these cancer cells. It also increases the incidences of the disease.

2. Blue light at night is contributing to blindness!

What I think was the most impressive part of his study is that he then looked at specific wavelengths or color of light at night to see which wavelength of light produced the greatest adverse effect, he found that the culprit was blue light. Blue light is very harmful to our eyes at night. We need blue light during the day, but we do not need blue light at night. It is very harmful. Unfortunately, in our society, we're being bombarded by blue light at night, especially with our government forcing us to use compact florescent lights at home; these emit a blue spectrum. Much healthier are the old-fashioned incandescent lights which give off a red spectrum. According to Dr. Abraham Haim, our greatest health risk right now is blue light at night, so I encourage all of you who have eye disease to reduce your exposure to blue light at night and use incandescent lights as much as possible. If you must work at the computer at night or if you use florescent lights, I would encourage you to purchase blue blocker glasses. They are available at drugstores, optical shops, or online.

Another study that confirms the importance of a dark environment at night was done with 100 patients who were given three milligrams of melatonin at night for a minimum of three nights to help them sleep. They were required to sleep in a totally dark room. The majority of patients who participated had a reduction in pathological macular changes. The daily use of three milligrams of melatonin seems to protect the retina and delay macular degeneration. My advice is to get a good night's sleep in a totally dark room; use a motion detector light if you need to get up to use the bathroom or a flashlight.

Ultraviolet light: friend or foe? Our main source of ultraviolet light as well as vitamin D is the sun. We recommend that everyone be tested for vitamin D levels, because just about everybody needs a supplement. I think our avoiding the sun for so long has contributed to ill health. Ultraviolet light is essential to our health, and lack of it may be a cause of macular degeneration because it has been proven that an important cellular layer of the macula needs low levels of ultraviolet light to regenerate.

Just about every eye doctor read and recalls a study done on monkeys that seemed to prove that UV light caused eye damage. It is such a flawed (not to mention cruel) study that Dr. Ott, who wrote the book about ultraviolet light and our health, stated, "This is much like having a group of people go into a blast furnace and become badly burned, and then concluding that heat is bad for the body."

The bottom line is that we do need ultraviolet light, but we need it in moderation. Personally, I no longer wear sunglasses. I feel that a moderate amount of ultraviolet light is essential to our health. You have to be careful if you've had cataract surgery and your lens has been removed; you do need sunglasses to protect your eye.

NEXT, I'M GOING TO TALK ABOUT VISION THERAPY. Vision is more than acuity. Many patients will have an improvement of their acuity when they finish our boot camp at the Wellness Center in Florida, but they may still struggle with reading. Functional vision is more important than acuity. Sometimes I'll see patients who are only able to read the first couple of lines on the eye chart, but they're able to function well. On the other hand, I have patients who are able to read the bottom line of the eye chart, and they're struggling to read. I think this whole idea of function is important, and many need vision training to use their eyes properly.

Dr. William Bates, a turn-of-the-century ophthalmologist, understood functional vision and the proper use of the eye. When I was in my medical residency, we learned to view Dr. Bates with great suspicion. Then I read the book, *The Art of Seeing*, by Aldous Huxley, a great science fiction writer, philosopher, and visionary. Huxley had horrible eyesight most of his life. At one time during his life, he had to read using braille. He went to different ophthalmology clinics throughout the country, and no one could help him.

Then he came across the work of Dr. Bates and underwent some of the therapies Dr. Bates talked about. They actually restored his vision, and he wrote *The Art of Seeing*, which discusses the Bates method in detail.

There's another book called *Relearning to See* by Tom Quackenbush, who has been a guest on my radio show. He discusses three elements of the Bates exercises: palming, swinging, and sunning.

Palming is a wonderful exercise where you cover your closed eyes with your cupped palms. Bates felt that this helped the eyes relax. By closing your eyes and covering them with your palms you're producing a very dark environment. While palming, do some deep breathing to help relax. Not only is this a type of meditative technique to help your eyes relax, but it also is a form of microcurrent because our bodies are an energetic system. Our hands and palms are known for emitting energy. Kirlian photography has shown that our palms emit a low level of electromagnetic energy. By putting our hands over our eyes, we are able to direct healing into our eyes.

Meir Schneider is a vision therapist in California who was born with congenital glaucoma and cataracts and was declared legally blind after several unsuccessful surgeries. He performed palming and sunning and, believe it or not, restored his vision. He now has a California driver's license and has written several books about the restoration of vision, including

Self-Healing: My Life and Vision.

Sunning, another healing technique from Dr. Bates, involves looking at the sun with your closed eyes while you move your head from side to side as though saying, "no." You'll see the image of the sun going across your retina.

For the longest time, I didn't accept this as a method of treatment. It wasn't until I read an article about how low-level laser therapy improves vision in patients with age-related macular degeneration that I appreciated sunning. The treatment involves shining the laser through closed eyelids. A large percentage of patients experienced improved vision. This was published in Germany in the *Photomedicine and Laser Surgery Journal* in 2008. After reading this article, I purchased a red laser. It's also called a cold laser. When my wife was treating her eyes, she made the comment that it was just like looking at the sun. I realized that Bates was right. You don't have to buy an expensive laser to get its benefits.

In our office, we use a device called the Nidek MP-1, which retrains the eye to use a new focus of fixation. When people with a macular scar try to read, their brain is trained to look straight ahead, and that scar tissue or blind spot is in the way. What this machine does is retrains the eye to pick up a new focal point of fixation which is away from the scar, so it results in improved functional vision.

HOMEOPATHY IS AN IMPORTANT PART OF MY PRACTICE. It is my favorite alternative modality, and, when it cured my asthma, I was hooked on alternative medicine. Many people think that Samuel Hahnemann was the first homeopath, but they are wrong. It was Moses, believe it or not. In the Bible, Exodus 23:20, "He took the calf which they had made and burnt it in the fire, ground it to powder, sprayed it upon the water and made the children of Israel drink it." This is exactly how we make our homeopathic remedies. If the source is a metal, we pulverize it, burn it, and mix it in water, and then we drink it. The really fascinating thing is that we know the calf was the golden calf, and gold is a homeopathic remedy that we use to treat depression and despair. Moses was acting as a homeopath for his people.

Homeopathy respects the wisdom of the body and understands its intelligence. When we develop a symptom or a disease, it is because our body needs the symptom to maintain homeostasis or balance. If you believe your body has wisdom, choose techniques that help it. Then it no longer need produce symptoms. Homeopaths are very interested in symptoms and their subtlety. If you have a high fever, the homeopathic doctor will give you a homeopathic medicine which, in a larger dose, causes a fever.

Traditional medicine treats with opposites. If you have a high fever, you're given something to lower your temperature. If you have asthma, you're given something to relax your lungs. When I was cured of my asthma, I was actually given a homeopathic remedy that, when given in large doses, causes asthma.

Here are some other examples. If you have watering and tearing in your eyes, the homeopathic doctor will give you homeopathic onion, *Allium cepa*, because those of you who have peeled an onion know that it causes watering in your eyes. If you have a lot of redness and swelling, perhaps from an insect bite, you're given the homeopathic remedy *Apis mellifica*, made from the honeybee. If you have swelling and hemorrhaging in your eye, you're given a remedy made from the rattlesnake because the rattlesnake's bite produces hemorrhage.

This is called the Law of Similars. A substance that causes symptoms in a healthy person will cure those symptoms in a sick person. For example, the plant *Belladonna*, when ingested, produces a fever, bright redness of the face, and a throbbing headache. If a patient has these symptoms, they're given homeopathic *Belladonna.*

The other thing I like about homeopathy is its capacity to treat a number of conditions, whether physical, mental, or emotional, at the same time. We look at the whole person. The treatment is individualized for each person also. If you have an eye problem, depression, arthritis, and indigestion, you will need a different homeopathic remedy than someone with macular degeneration, high blood pressure, heart disease, and maybe a lot of anger.

Some of my best successes in treating patients have been using homeopathy. This is something that we do at the Healing the Eye & Wellness Center. I encourage everyone to explore homeopathy; find a homeopathic doctor in your area and receive homeopathic treatment because, not only can it help your general health, it can also be a tremendous help to your vision.

3. What treatment that reversed San Snead's vision loss can help you?

Microcurrent is one of our most successful treatments at the Healing the Eye & Wellness Center. This is a technique that improves blood flow, stimulates cellular activity, can remove and reduce scar tissue, reduces inflammation, and also has a neuroprotective effect. I have been using it for some years, and, over 15 years ago, I treated Sam Snead for his macular degeneration. He had great improvement in his vision. In exchange, he gave me golf lessons. Everyone asks what Sam told me about my golf game. He watched me hit a couple of buckets of balls and examined my swing from different angles. He came up to me, put his arm around me, and said, "Dr. Kondrot, here's what I want you to do. I want you to cut back for a year, and then just give up the game." I followed his advice. I cut back for a year. Now am so busy on the ranch and working at the Wellness Center that I just don't have any time for golf.

It always upsets me when a patient asks his/her eye doctor whether microcurrent can help and the eye doctor says, "Absolutely not. There have been no good studies to show that it can benefit your eye." I have to laugh because if that same patient asked the eye doctor, "If I could improve blood flow to my eye, stimulate cellular activity, and remove scar tissue, would it help me?" The answer, of course, is yes.

There have been many studies that show that microcurrent does these things. There are very few studies that show that it actually does it for the eye, but I believe that if there are good animal studies and studies in orthopedic medicine, plastic surgery, and transplant medicine, that prove it works on those parts of the body, it should work with the eye. I have done some studies using microcurrent on eye disease. I published a report in the *Townsend Letter* for physicians in 2002 describing my early experience. There have also been publications on microcurrent and the treatment of retinitis pigmentosa, a study done about microcurrent reducing intraocular pressure, and a study showing that microcurrent has a neuroprotective effect.

The United States Cycling Team routinely uses microcurrent for their sore muscles and injuries. A few years ago my wife and I ran the Marine Corps marathon. After the race, we were extremely sore; I could barely walk. A 30-minute application of microcurrent fully restored me. I couldn't believe that the inflammation causing my soreness was almost completely gone.

The early machines were rather crude. The MicroStim 100 is the first machine that I used, and we used it to treat the acupuncture points around the eye. This machine was limited because we only had four frequencies and one channel.

Why are the frequencies important? Every tissue has a unique frequency or vibration. What we want to do is match the frequency of the microcurrent to the tissue. When you match them, you get good results. It is similar to having two tuning forks that are each vibrating at a C-sharp frequency, resonance. We have found that by using tissue-specific microcurrent frequency we are increasing the effects of this treatment.

The machine that we're now using is an Inspirstar machine. This is a programmable machine with five specific programs. With it, we are able to give a patient a customized treatment plan to use at home. After a patient participates in the Healing the Eye & Wellness Center program, we load their specific settings into the microcurrent machine, and then they take the machine home for further treatment. The current machine is really easy to use and has capacity that allows us to vary the frequency as needed for the patient.

I am often asked why our machines are so expensive when you can buy a microcurrent machine on eBay for under $100. The machines on eBay are not microcurrent. Many of them are TENS units, which have a much higher current. It has been found that the lower current is better at stimulating healing and reducing inflammation than high currents. Dr.

Cheng did a study that demonstrated that a current less than 500 micro amps is best for improving cellular activity.

In addition to your eye, we can treat selected parts of your body with microcurrent. For example we may put it over your abdomen to treat your liver and kidneys to detoxify as well as reduce stress.

I am participating in a microcurrent research project with the Department of Ophthalmology at the University of Rome. This study is measuring the effects of microcurrent on an animal model of macular degeneration. My wife and I spent two months in Rome developing the research project. We plan to go back to Rome to finish it. It is very exciting that a major university center is interested in microcurrent.

Many of us are unaware that we are experiencing current all the time. The earth's magnetic field is referred to as the fifth element. It was discovered that when the Soviet cosmonauts came back from space, although they were given the four elements of oxygen, water, excellent nutrition, and ultraviolet light, they were very weak and debilitated. Scientists discovered that this is because they had been deprived of the fifth element, the Earth's magnetic field. Over the last 165 years, scientists have determined that the Earth's magnetic field is declining in strength. Today the magnetic field is measured at about 0.5 gauss. Four thousand years ago, it was 5 gauss. That's a decrease of 90%. Just like the Soviet cosmonauts sickened when they were deprived of the magnetic field, we are suffering from its reduced strength. Rubber-soled shoes also contribute to our being out of touch with the magnetic field. Years ago, all shoes were leather. Now, more and more shoes are rubber, which is a powerful insulator. We are no longer grounded to the Earth.

A phenomenal book called *Earthing*, written by alternative doctor Stephen Sinatra, suggests that earthing or grounding is a very important health practice. To experience it, remove your shoes and socks and walk on the ground. Doing this increases your magnetic connection with the Earth and charges the electromagnetic field in your body. Dr. Sinatra reports on many cases of chronic disease improving simply by doing earthing.

At the Florida Wellness Center, we also offer a number of specialized therapies such as chelation, oxidative therapies, and hyperbaric oxygen. These are all geared to detoxification. The best way to remove lead is by chelation therapies, administered by intravenous, rectal, topical, or oral means. Intravenous is best because 100% of the chelating agent is absorbed in your body. With the rectal treatment, only 25% is absorbed. Topical is primarily used for treating autistic children who may have mercury toxicity. Of course, oral is less effective. Oral can be helpful if it's combined with the rectal. If IV administration is not possible, we recommend using a combination of rectal suppositories and oral detox.

OXIDATIVE THERAPIES are a very powerful way of stimulating the body to heal. Ozone is a highly reactive form of oxygen that dramatically increases oxygen concentrations in your body. It stimulates regeneration and healing and triggers a lot of beneficial neuroendocrine chemical reactions in the body that are essential for regaining your health.

One type of ozone therapy is autohemotherapy, where we actually combine the ozone with blood that we have drawn and then re-infuse it. A newer treatment that we're investigating is rectal insufflation. This has been developed by Silvia Menendez, a Cuban researcher, and offers many benefits. She has treated thousands of patients with eye problems, and 90% have improved. I favor treatments that patients can do at home, and rectal insufflation is one that you can continue doing at home if you buy the necessary equipment.

Stem cell treatment of eye disease has received some attention. I have studied this method and am not using it currently since I am not sure of its results. Doctors who do use stem cells are very cautious about reducing inflammation and removing toxins in their patients. It is also necessary to improve oxygenation and eliminate heavy metals. I have found that if you do these things, your body is naturally going to heal without actually using stem cell therapy. At this point, my work focuses on microcurrent, oxidative treatments, and light therapy, and the results are much better than what is achieved through more conventional methods.

I intend to continue to research and develop methods to prevent, arrest, and, when possible, cure vision problems. I encourage anyone with eye disease to refuse to accept the dire predictions of conventional medicine and to begin a course of healing, using as many of the methods I have described as possible. There is always hope.

....

EDWARD KONDROT, MD, MD (H), CCH, DHT
President of the Arizona Homeopathic and Integrative Medical Association
Clinic Director of the American Medical College of Homeopathy
Host of *Healthy Vision Talk Radio*
Director of the Florida Wellness Center
31242 Amberlea Road
Dade City, FL 33523
(800)430-9328
www.HealingTheEye.com
info@HealingTheEye.com

James Lemire, MD

OCALA, FLORIDA

Interviewed December 2, 2013

1. **Jimmy was told that there was nothing that could be done; today, he's alive and well and running on the beach.**

2. **With my treatment to reverse deteriorated cartilage, surgery can be avoided in many cases.**

3. **This ancient treatment helps deal with chronic illnesses of today including allergies, sinusitis, bronchitis, inflammation, and fatigue.**

DR. KONDROT: I refer to Dr. Lemire as a Renaissance practitioner because he's doing so many eclectic things in his practice. Before we talk about the uniqueness of your practice or what makes you a Renaissance practitioner, please tell me a little bit about your background and training. You're like most of us. You didn't really begin doing alternative or integrative treatments. You started out as a conventional medical doctor, right?

DR. LEMIRE: That's correct. I had an early interest in medicine. I had a brother with cerebral palsy who was taken care of by an osteopathic physician years ago. I went to medical school at Tulane University, a very traditional medical school in New Orleans. I had a natural affinity for family practice. Unfortunately, Tulane didn't really nurture that. They didn't have a family practice residency program until years after I left, but I always remembered our own family doctor who introduced me to family practice, particularly from an alternative view. I didn't know at that time that they called them "alternative." I earned a traditional medical degree from Tulane. Then, I did a three-year family practice residency in Grand Rapids, Michigan, and then I did 20 years of the traditional family practice from cradle to grave. I did 500 deliveries and took care of the elderly.

My interest in getting out of that mold started when I taught sports medicine and met many osteopathic physicians and began learning about osteopathic manipulation and how the spine is so important to health. I began exploring diet, exercise, and nutrition, which were critical to the health of athletes. I was a volunteer Olympic team physician in 1992 and took care of world-class athletes.

After I got tired of shoveling snow in Michigan, I moved to Ocala, Florida, and began looking at how to incorporate diet, exercise, and nutrition into my program. I went to the American College for Advancement in Medicine meeting, where I met my mentor and our mutual good friend, Dr. Garry Gordon, the father of chelation therapy. He introduced me to chelation therapy and the world of alternative medicine. My life has never been the same since. Dr. Gordon introduced me to Bruce Shelton, a family physician and a classically trained homeopath. I began to receive training in homeopathy and to incorporate those skills.

A chiropractor by the name of John Brimhall worked out of Dr. Gordon's and Dr. Shelton's offices. He expanded his practice and is now world-renowned for the Brimhall Method of chiropractic, which uses applied kinesiology to determine imbalances in muscles and how people respond to medicines and supplements.

Last year, I, along with two others, wrote a book called *The Ultimate Guide to Natural Health, the Premier Handbook for Natural Health in the 21st Century* with chapters by some of our mutual friends, Dr. Brimhall, Dr. Gordon, and Dr. Lee Cowden, who does a lot with Lyme disease. You also know Dr. Stephen Sinatra, who wrote a chapter on earthing and grounding; he, in fact, introduced me to energy medicine. Dr. Gordon also introduced me to Dr. Robert Rowen, a good friend of yours who trained me in ozone therapy, so I've added ozone therapy. We use it for chronically ill patients and for helping to repair joints.

As I began to apply all of those skills into my family medicine practice, I began to see that there was a way to integrate all of traditional medicine and all of the alternative methods I was learning. We just call it good medicine! Good medicine is using the right technique or form for the individual patient. I've continued to expand that notion. I met people from the Institute for Functional Medicine and began learning that there were people looking at disease from a sense of what the underlying cause is.

Traditional medicine, for example, would say that hypertension is a disease. We, on the other hand, would look at it as a symptom. Maybe that person has been exposed to heavy metals. Many of our clients older than 65 have been exposed to heavy metals, particularly lead, their whole lives. That might be a key component to developing a treatment plan. If we remove the lead or control the lead in their systems, we may control the high blood pressure without having to treat the end symptom, which is the blood pressure itself. That's how I've taken this approach to integrative medicine. We now call it functional medicine.

These are advanced techniques that complement what the Eastern training and Western training do, and we've incorporated that into what we do in our unique practice. My wife is a board-certified occupational therapist, and she does acupuncture and cranial sacral work. She also is now doing all of our nutritional work. We have added a chiropractor to our staff. We have two massage therapists. One does a Tai Chi type of massage, and one is traditional but has added Reiki. We have integrated many of the energy medicine techniques into our practice.

We then went on and looked at the changes in medicine and how to provide services alternatively in the future. Even with the changes in insurance, we want to have all of these services available for everyone. So, for the last six years, I have taken courses through the Institute for Functional Medicine. In September of this year, I took the boards for certification in functional medicine. I'm in one of the first groups of physicians certified in functional medicine.

DR. KONDROT: I admire you first for your strong background as a family practitioner, cradle to grave. That's what I think makes a really good physician. We need that life experience dealing with the different aspects of health. Then there's your experience with sports medicine and osteopathy. That wide background enables one to get a deeper understanding of the body and understand what true health is. Could you please explain your approach to evaluating a patient who comes to you with a particular health problem? How is your approach unique?

DR. LEMIRE: I would choose a patient named Jimmy. He's 58. He was a missionary to Guatemala and was exposed to a lot of heavy chemicals and pesticides. He developed a heart issue and had to retire. He came back to this country and ended up having a stent put in. We looked at the EKGs and the heart catherization reports. He was found to have cardiomyopathy, which is a significant weakening of the heart. Because he had no insurance, he could not afford to have a defibrillator put into his heart. That's the only way they thought he would survive.

1. Jimmy was told that there was nothing that could be done; today, he's alive and well and running on the beach.

He came to us having had all of the traditional blood work, EKGs, and heart catheterizations. They told him there was nothing else they could do for him and to go home and die. We did kinesiology and energetically looked at him and found that he was very weak; his adrenals and hormones were weak. We did some confirming studies to see that his hormones were very low. We did a heavy metal challenge; we know that people with cardiomyopathy have about a 200% higher chance of having mercury or lead in their bodies. That's what we found, so that gave us a different direction.

You and I and our alternative colleagues always want to give people hope. Patients come to us saying they were told to go home and die. We are their last resort. They have to have hope. Well, we gave Jimmy hope. We started doing chelation therapy where we removed the heavy metals intravenously. We started doing nutritional work. We put him on magnesium, ribose, CoQ10, and L-Carnitine, which are the things we know nutritionally strengthen the heart. We used kinesiology to muscle test what types of supplements he needed and how often, and balanced a program for him. We did the traditional testosterone studies and found that heavy metals blocked his testosterone, so we started him on testosterone shots.

The last piece of the puzzle before we did his IVs was that we did pulse electromagnetic field therapy. Dr. Gordon introduced me to that method two years ago; it uses a wave of electromagnetic therapy that strengthens the heart from the inside out. It strengthens the heart without the exercise. The most important study

showed that he had an ejection fraction of only 15%. Normal ejection fraction for a healthy male would be 50% to 60%. We traditionally know from the studies that anybody below 20% is basically a cardiac cripple, and he really was. He could only wear sweat pants because his legs were swollen. His heart was congested and he had fluid. He could only walk from the house to the mailbox, and he got short of breath doing that.

We were treating him three times a week with a combination of hormones and nutrition. Then we removed the heavy metals with chelation therapy and strengthened his heart with pulse electromagnetic field treatments.

We got him off the heavy grains he was eating. Two books, *Grain Brain* by Dr. David Perlmutter and *Wheat Belly* by Dr. William Davis, tell us we need to get off grains. Wheat is genetically modified and creates a lot of inflammation.

He began to get up and get around. The process has taken about a year and a half. We have a pre-photo of him just sitting in his house. He was edematous, swollen, and really unable to do anything. My wife just got a new photo of him, looking fit, trim, 30 pounds lighter, and in the pink of health. We repeated his studies and modified and adjusted his medicine with our applied kinesiology, but we also found that his ejection fraction is now 33%. We basically more than doubled it.

The man now has a great quality of life using a combination of all the things that we do, such as IV nutrition, removing heavy metals, and replenishing his hormones and nutrition. Here was a man who had extensive weakening of his heart. We looked at the causes, taking out and treating each of those, like the nutritional deficiency, strengthening the heart with the pulse electromagnetic therapy, removing the inflammatory foods in his diet, and then restoring his testosterone level using bio-organic hormonal creams that I learned about from Dr. Jonathan Wright many years ago.

We put all of these techniques together. Functional medicine looks at the underlying cause of disease and then treats it. We still used traditional drugs to help with strengthening his heart, but we also did all of the things we do naturally, as well as the treatments like IV chelation and pulse electromagnetic field therapy.

And so, we have changed a man who was told to go home and die. His wife was really pleased when we saw her a week ago. She said, "You've given me the best Thanksgiving present I could have. I'm really thankful that I have my husband back, and we are able to do things again." He's alive and well and running on the beach in the Bahamas on their first vacation in almost two years. Those are the kinds of results that we see with functional medicine.

All of these functional medicine techniques can be used for many illnesses and chronic diseases because our bodies have been so worn down by poor diet, poor nutrition, and the environment that people live in. We all are toxic. We are

having good results with eye disease, also.

I'm in the sundown of my career at this point, yet I've had many newborns in my practice since I've been in Florida. The reason is because we offer the same thing to newborns and their families: we offer them choices in health from a very young age, choices that work.

DR. KONDROT: The question I'd like to ask is, "Where does traditional Western medicine fall short?" I'm sure this guy with cardiomyopathy saw some of the top cardiologists and was on the latest petrochemical drug to stimulate his heart, and yet traditional Western medicine gave up. I see the same situation in my ophthalmology practice. Patients can be under excellent care and have the latest surgery, but they just don't get better. What do you think is the missing ingredient?

DR. LEMIRE: The traditional cardiologists in this case just focused on medication. We become ill and there's a pill. That's what we're trying to get away from and look at the whole patient. They have gotten away from looking at the whole patient and how the drugs affect the whole patient, sometimes adversely.

DR. KONDROT: Can you tell us the treatments that you really enjoy doing and that you feel have a lot of versatility in your practice? What are the top three treatments?

DR. LEMIRE: It's hard to pick three specific

treatments, but I'll list the things I do a lot. We do IV nutritional therapy to take out heavy metals. The Environmental Work Group, which is an organization in New York, has done studies of how toxic we are. Albert Einstein College of Medicine has a detox program that costs about $10,000. They look at 425 known heavy metals, pesticides, and toxins like DDT that are found in our bodies. They measure them and give the results. The average American has about 325. What that means is that everybody in this country is toxic and we need to be able to do something to detoxify.

It's not just our generation, but it's our children, grandchildren, and great grandchildren. The Environmental Work Group did a fetal cord blood study. They analyzed the blood from ten healthy infants' cords. They found 278 known toxins.

One of the reasons I'm seeing more children now is because we're encouraging people to detoxify their children. We all need detoxification therapies that take out heavy metals. Dr. Gordon said the first thing his mother told him was that he had to get the lead out. He has been doing that ever since.

Dr. Gordon uses both IVs and orals because he needs to have a balance of continuous detoxification. We do both form, also. With all the newborns and children I'm seeing, we have to incorporate the mindset of detoxification from birth. That's why parents have to have a choice when they're giving their kids vaccinations. Families have been so browbeaten by the traditional medical system, telling them that if you don't give your child his Hepatitis B shot in the first 24 hours of life, you're a bad parent. You know and the public needs to know that Hepatitis B is passed on sexually, so a child will never really be exposed to Hepatitis B until he's of an age to be sexually active. Yet, we're doing that in the first 24 hours of life when the child's immune system is just beginning to develop. We have to have sanity in the immunization program. Shots can be postponed. We can make safer vaccines that don't contain mercury or aluminum, which are known neurotoxins.

Those of us who receive Dr. Gordon's regular newsletters and emails have learned that there can be vaccines that aren't harmful, but we are still giving harmful vaccine, prepared with mercury, to children, particularly the flu shot.

Another area that I like to work with is bioidentical hormones. Suzanne Somers is one of the pioneers in promoting this. She wrote a book called *Knockout*. Our friends Dr. Jonathan Wright and Dr. Garry Gordon have chapters in it. She's trying to make women aware of the natural hormones that can balance their bodies. After a woman who has had a hysterectomy goes through menopause, she has lost the ability to balance her hormones.

That's actually a series I'm giving in my office right now where I focus on one hormone for a month. I did the thyroid last month. This month, we're going to be covering the adrenals. Replacing hormones bioidentically and balancing them is such an important key to health. You and I were trained to give a woman one dose of a synthetic estrogen and progestin; one size fits all. We know that approach has had bad results. I think that using bioidentical hormones is very helpful for balancing both men and women.

We see the low T commercials on TV for men. This gentleman we took care of with the weakened heart needed testosterone. We used bioidentical testosterone to raise his levels up to a reasonable level. He had to have it as a supplement because all the heavy metals were blocking his own ability to produce it.

The third technique involves hands. I learned manipulation therapy while teaching and taking courses with the osteopathic physicians at Michigan State. I taught them sports medicine, and they taught me how to do manipulative therapy.

The knee is a structure that deteriorates with the wear and tear of the activities of life. The problem is that we eat poorly. We don't ingest enough omega-3 fatty acids and don't give the proper nourishment to the knee, and then we overuse it and it breaks down. I used to do a lot of cortisone injections. However, when I was working with Olympic athletes, they can't have cortisone because it eliminates them from competition. We started using prolotherapy, which was designed 34 years ago. Even C. Everett Koop learned the technique, and he was the Surgeon General of the United States. When his neck was deteriorating somebody taught him prolotherapy.

2. With my treatment to reverse deteriorated cartilage, surgery can be avoided in many cases.

I began using prolotherapy, which is a reconstructive therapy using a homeopathic substance along with sugar water injected into the knee to help it to heal. When somebody goes to an orthopedic surgeon or a traditional surgeon and are told, "You actually show bone on bone. The only thing for you to do is have an artificial knee." Some people do need an artificial knee, but we now have a way to actually reverse that deteriorated cartilage; it's called ozone. It's a technique we use for prolozone therapy. You put ozone into the knee. Dr. Frank Shallenberger has studies reversing the deterioration of the joint so that people are not forced into having a total knee replacement. Any joint can have this treatment. I do multiple types of joints.

I've also learned prolozone therapy. The Heel Company calls it bioacupuncture because you're putting Heel-type products or homeopathic remedies into the joint. My goal is to not only slow the deterioration but also actually reverse it. It's a great thing to have somebody say, "I'm scheduled for knee surgery. Do I have to have it?" I say, "Let's try this." I have many cases now where people never had to have surgery.

Some of the traditional orthopedic surgeons I've met are beginning to listen. They don't want to have the unsuccessful result of somebody coming back where the surgery was perfect but the results were not, and the people have continued pain. I'm educating our local orthopedic surgeons to test for titanium allergies, just as we do for other allergies. Maybe an allergic patient needs the new zirconium implants instead of titanium. Some surgeons are looking at doing some serum plasma injections or stem cells, which is another whole broad area. We've just begun to touch the surface with our good friend Dr. Dave Steenblock.

DR. KONDROT: This is fascinating. I can attest to the prolozone therapy. After hiking for ten days in the Grand Canyon, I developed tendinitis, which was not responsive to heat or stretching. After just one ozone injection, I had my normal leg back. It can be very dramatic.

I would like you to talk about what I think is your most interesting treatment, one based on an ancient practice. I've used this treatment twice with just amazing results. Tell us about it.

DR. LEMIRE: We use the Himalayan salt therapy. Modern history dates it back to Poland. In 1843, a Polish physician, Felik Boczkowski, noted that workers in the salt mines were unlike any other mine workers he had ever seen. They didn't have black lung and respiratory problems.

3. This ancient treatment helps deal with the chronic illnesses of today including allergies, sinusitis, bronchitis, inflammation, and fatigue.

Salt is known to have antibacterial and anti-inflammatory properties. In Europe, they began opening spas in the salt caves. Today it's very popular. Halotherapy is another word for salt therapy. Spas have been opened throughout Eastern Europe, Russia, and Canada. It has spread into Australia and New Zealand, and now it's in the United States. There are probably 45 to 60 Himalayan salt rooms in the United States. There are other salt rooms that use sea salt. We like the Himalayan salt because it has 84 minerals in it that help replenish the trace elements in our body.

We have created what we call our salt cave. It has 9,000 pounds of salt on the walls, the ceiling, and the floor. The person sits in the cave for a 45-minute session. They come out refreshed and their nasal passages are clear. This helps with many different types of problems. It's effective for treating respiratory problems such as asthma and bronchitis and skin conditions such as eczema and psoriasis.

One of the differences between Himalayan salt and table salt is that Himalayan salt has a color to it, from pink to red to dark crimson with white flecks in it. It comes from the Himalayan mountain range; we order ours from Pakistan. It hasn't been processed. A lot of the other salts, particularly the sea salts that come from the Mediterranean or the Caribbean, have to be processed in order to make them.

We use salt lamps, too. People can buy them, bring them home, and put them by their computers, in their bedroom, or their living room. A salt lamp generates negative ions, which help to purify the air, remove the pollutants and bacteria, and just create a healthy climate within their home.

Asthma is a common respiratory condition in this country. People get inflammation of the lungs and the lungs narrow with what we call bronchospasm. Those people get really short of breath. When these people breathe in the aerosol salt particles, the negative charge helps to break down the mucus and has a very strong anti-inflammatory, anti-allergy, and purifying effect on the respiratory systems of people with asthma. Children do really well. They come in wheezing and short of breath. After a treatment, they go out of there breathing much easier. Parents can buy a salt lamp to put in their room for treatments at home.

Salt has been used for a long time to preserve meat; it helps to reduce the harmful bacteria and other pathogenic microorganisms. Those negative ions, too, help to reduce inflammation. In Florida, we have mold issues because of the heavy humidity. Salt helps reduce the irritation from the mold. Arizona probably doesn't have much of a mold problem, but Arizona has a lot of allergens because of the bloom in the desert. For people

with seasonal allergies, the Himalayan salt therapy reduces swelling in the nasal passages, helping drain and unblock the sinuses, and then people can really breathe more easily.

The salt works by staying in your respiratory tract, allowing the mucus to flow away from the sinuses, allowing people to naturally cough things up. That's one of the reasons that allergic people have coughing spells. The thick mucus is so tenacious that they can't get it out of the sinuses. How often have you talked to people who have chronic postnasal drainage? This is a great therapy for people with chronic respiratory problems.

As functional medicine doctors we know that milk is one of the biggest culprits because it increases mucus. We were never designed to drink milk long-term. Another culprit is wheat, which is so genetically changed since when we were kids, that many more people are wheat sensitive. They might not have true celiac disease, but they have a lot of asthma and allergy symptoms because they're eating wheat that has been so processed and genetically modified that their bodies can no longer handle it. Our treatments will help open up their lungs and breathe more easily.

Then there are skin conditions. People who have inflammatory problems with their skin, such as eczema or psoriasis, notice an improvement in just one or two sessions in the salt room. It reduces the inflammatory blebs, gets the redness out, and helps heal the skin.

Remind people how good they feel when they are at the beach. They've been breathing the salt air. They've been getting the moisture in the air and it's like a vacation. Forty-five minutes in our salt room is like a two-day vacation in Tahiti.

....

JAMES LEMIRE, MD
Lemire Clinic
11115 SW 93rd Ct. Rd, Suite 600,
Ocala, FL 34481
(352)291-9459
www.LemireClinic.com
www.HimalayanSaltRoomOcala.com

Ruth Tan Lim, MD MD(H), FAAP FAAARAM

MESA, ARIZONA

Interviewed May 26, 2013

1. **Breastfeeding mothers have more success when they eat for their own as well as their baby's blood type.**

2. **My approach to immunizations is to go slow and low.**

3. **The entire hormonal system needs to be balanced before replacement therapy can be effective.**

DR. KONDROT: Dr. Ruth Tan Lim is a practicing physician and board-certified in pediatrics, anti-aging, and regenerative medicine. It seems like she does it all from young children to aging adults.

She's a licensed homeopathic doctor and on the board of the Arizona Homeopathic and Integrated Medical Association with me. We're working diligently to help educate the Arizona community, and, for that matter the United States, on the benefits of alternative and integrative medicine. Please share how you got interested in medicine and integrative techniques in your practice.

DR. LIM: I came from the University of

Singapore. That was where I graduated. I came to Arizona in 1979 about 34 years ago. In 1996, I looked at the practice of medicine, which was my daily job, and the whole medical industry, and I felt I needed to rethink and reinvent it for myself with more avenues of approach helping patients on their healing. I decided to research integrating my practice with other modalities because when we practice conventional medicine, we use a lot of pharmaceuticals. I thought my toolbox was kind of limited, and I needed to really expand. That was when I started my own journey of education, motivation, and transformation.

Of course, it's been really beneficial not only for me but also for my staff and certainly for my patients. I usually see patients from newborns, children, young adults, and their family members who are interested in integrative modalities. The family members see the value of integrative modalities, and many want a consultation so they can better function as they go into the more mature years of their lives. That's how I got started. I just had to think outside the box.

DR. KONDROT: Let's talk a little bit about your pediatric practice. What do you think is the biggest challenge to keeping children healthy?

DR. LIM: Over the 33 years since I've been settled in Arizona practicing pediatrics, I think we have a bigger problem today with nutrition. Metabolic syndrome is really big. As I see all these kids, they're becoming chunkier.

Related to this are problems in mental cognition and learning. There are actually a lot of mood disorders. Those are probably the top three. It's the metabolic, which is their weight, then their mental, which is their memory, and then their mood. That's what I think is facing children today.

DR. KONDROT: Let's start by talking a little bit about nutrition because this not only affects children but also adults. When you see a child, or for that matter an adult, what advice do you give in terms of nutrition?

1. Breastfeeding mothers have more success when they eat for their own as well as their baby's blood type.

DR. LIM: I see newborns. One of the most common newborn problems is feeding. I ask parents, especially the mother, what their blood type is. I always make sure the hospital does the baby's blood type. Maternal nutrition is important for breastfeeding mothers. Following the blood type diet does help to reduce problems of feeding in the newborn such as colic, gas, and fussiness. I ask the mother to learn about and follow the *Eat Right for Your Blood Type* diet. It seems to help a lot, especially when they have a really colicky baby. Avoiding wheat and dairy is often beneficial. If you're a Type O like me and reduce your wheat intake and your dairy intake, the overall health is better. Many times when we do this little adjustment, the baby seems to do much better. We also start the infant on probiotics. Sometimes we use formula to supplement the babies. We try not to use cow's milk-based formula.

The other thing we see in pediatrics are allergies. This is linked to leaky gut and dysbiosis. As children get a little older, we see infections, allergies, and a lot of related things in the airways. We do see a lot of different diagnoses such as allergic rhinitis, bronchitis, reactive airway disease, and asthma. If the child is on too many antibiotics, I evaluate them to make sure they are really needed. We start them on gut repair, using probiotics and glutamine.

I do their lab work and found this very useful in children who have a lot of respiratory illness, especially kids with asthma. Most of them are very low in vitamin D and magnesium. Many times when I start them on vitamin D3 over a few months and bring them up to more optimum levels, their asthma improves. Also I encourage families to use almond milk which is a good source for magnesium.

Usually in children with learning problems and ADHD, we don't use pharmaceuticals. We do nutritional assessments and teach parents to use non-processed foods and foods without coloring. That's more of a natural, healthy diet. There seems to be improvement. We also use homeopathic remedies and encourage families to consult a developmental specialist and neurologist for a complete evaluation.

When we do the lab work on ADHD children, many times we find that their iron is a little low. When we start using simple low-dose iron supplements, they seem to do very well. These are just some of the scenarios that I see day to day.

DR. KONDROT: I guess you're not a really big advocate of the commercial baby food.

DR. LIM: No. I encourage all moms to breastfeed. They can do that until the mom and the baby want to quit. If they

are very depressed and have other things going or are very stressed and their milk production is down, then I do encourage them to supplement. I do recommend that the breastfeeding moms continue their prenatal vitamins and drink a lot of fluids and take adequate protein and vegetables in their diet.

We also recommend the breast milk banks. Some mothers donate their extra breast milk for other babies. We still work on as natural an approach as possible.

I do teach parents how to shop, though. I think shopping is very important because sometimes they just go to the supermarket and buy everything. They need to really spend their time shopping carefully, reading labels carefully, and not buying processed food.

They need to eat simple things like from the days of their great-grandparents or grandparents so that everything is more plant-based. I support plant-based diets. I think that's really a good key to start off with so there will not be too many additives or dyes in the diet and to work on a more balanced diet with refills on vegetables and fruits.

DR. KONDROT: Dr. Ruth, I wonder if you could give us your opinion on the overuse of antibiotics. Then we'll talk a little bit about immunizations. Are they necessary in children? First, let's talk about antibiotics.

DR. LIM: Every day I have parents say, "I would like the child not to receive any more antibiotics," because they've been to different physicians who may prescribe antibiotics freely, even for a cold.

The way I approach all this is depends on the information and the evaluation. I make sure we do not miss a treatable infection. If I get a case of sore throat where the tonsils are inflamed, we do a rapid culture. If it is positive for strep throat, we'll use a good short, simple five-day regimen rather than a ten-day regimen of antibiotics. It has been shown that recurrent streptococcal infection is related to the PANDAS, which is Pediatric Autoimmune Neuropsychiatric Disease Associated with Streptococcal Infection, and some children manifest concentration and learning problems later on.

However, if the child does not have a strep throat and is stable, I tell the mother that the process of all this so-called infection or inflammation could be viral. Fifty percent could be viral. Maybe 35% or 40% could be bacterial. Maybe 10% could be something else.

Normally, I recommend that the parents put the child on probiotics, give plenty of fluids, and start them on vitamin C. We also use some homeopathic remedies to restore and rebalance and reduce inflammation. I like to use Galium Oral Drops by HEEL. It is one of the top anti-viral products. I also use a lot of vitamin C. I prefer the powdered form because just one teaspoon can give you almost 4,000 milligrams. That really helps the mitochondria of the cells so that the cells are healthier and can handle the infection better.

At the same time, I follow the techniques from Chinese medicine. If you're sick, you should eat more of a plant-based diet and keep your liver healthy which can help healing.

Some of these techniques seem to be pretty effective. If I do have to treat a child with congestion, I suggest conventional allopathic decongestants like hydroxyzine. Sometimes, I use a promethazine for their cough. I also use drainage and cough remedies like Guna Noni. I like Astragalus tinctures, especially in the wintertime, to build up lung immunity. I also use Echinacea tinctures and vitamin D3. They have drops for babies that seem to help with bronchial conditions.

If a child has a very significant infection, then I will use conventional allopathic treatment and write a prescription.

I think overuse of antibiotics is a real concern because when children go to the emergency room or urgent care, sometimes the doctors are not sure what they have, so they often prescribe antibiotics.

The other factor is the parents. They may have a very heavy schedule and are very busy. They're worried that the school or the babysitter will keep calling them. Many times they *want* antibiotics, but I try to encourage them not to be dependent on them.

DR. KONDROT: I like the approach of looking at the underlying cause because

I think the overuse of antibiotics is such a serious problem in our country, especially in kids. You factor in the strength of the body and the liver and change the diet. Now let's talk about a more controversial subject. That's this whole idea of immunizations.

DR. LIM: I've been a physician now for 44 years. When I was in medical school, we gave immunizations. In the United States, we have a very good immunization program. However, I think some feel that too many vaccines are given at one time. In other countries, they phase it in more gradually.

Immunization is the best gift that we have given to humanity. Look at all the diseases, especially polio, we are preventing. I think polio is a devastating disease.

I'm a Rotarian and support Rotary's effort to eradicate polio. We've been doing this for almost 30 years. We are partnering with the Bill Gates Foundation that gave us about $300 million to try to eradicate polio.

2. My approach to immunizations is to go slow and low.

I take what they call the both sides approach regarding immunizations. In other words, I go slow and low. I see people who come to my practice bringing their children along with a schedule from Dr. Bob Sears. I'll order that, and we'll do that. Dr. Sears' schedule is, of course, go slow and go low.

I would say the most important immunization is DTaP: diphtheria, tetanus, and pertussis. Do you know that with pertussis there's no permanent immunity? Theoretically, a one-day-old baby can catch the disease. The younger the child is, the more devastating it is. If an adult has a cough for more than 72 hours, they'd better be sure that they are not a carrier of pertussis.

It's very well known that the school bus driver and the older grandparents are all carriers of whooping cough. Nowadays because we have to protect the next generation, we're even offering DTaP immunization to young childbearing age parents, both for the mom and the dad, because we want to protect the babies.

I've seen all these diseases when I practiced in Singapore many years ago. We had a very significant immunization program there that changed the face of treatment. It was amorphous influenza Type B.

When I came to Arizona in the 1970s or 1980s, I would admit about 12 cases of bacterial meningitis a year to the hospital. Nowadays, we don't see it anymore because of the good protection and herd immunity with the vaccine for Haemophilus influenzae Type B. They give it from 0 to 15 months, four doses at different times. We've almost wiped out this illness. This also goes for pneumococcal disease.

That's why it's very important to be wise in choosing a schedule that we call go slow and go low. In other words, you don't have to take so many at one time.

DR. KONDROT: Now we're going to switch focus a little bit and talk about the other end of the spectrum, the aging. I really admire you, Dr. Lim, for managing both ends of the spectrum from the very young to aging patients. Let's talk a little bit about your anti-aging and regenerative practice.

DR. LIM: In 1996, I told you I had to revamp my own career. I went ahead and took all the classes and courses that were offered by the American Academy of Anti-Aging and Regenerative Medicine.

I found out in my own practice with the biggest kids ages 16 to 20 that their brain function is really a bit sluggish. Many times they would tell me, "Dr. Lim, I study so hard. I went in to take the test. I got brain fog and could not remember," or "My concentration is really not good."

I've learned from the American Academy of Anti-Aging fellowship on the brain segment that you have ways of keeping your brain cells healthy. The most important thing that I started to research is what the Linus Pauling Institute on health and medicine teaches: It is function, not age, and depends on what the brain is exposed to during the formative or learning years.

Gradually, I started to use homeopathic remedies even in younger people to help them with their memory. I like to use *Baryta carbonica*, for example.

I also use *cerebrum compositum*, and it really improved my high school and college-aged patients' memories and concentration.

The other thing to look at is nutrition. Many times their diets are not good. I started to do other research and found out that Linus Pauling Institute recommends acetyl L-carnitine as a very good molecule for the brain. In fact, lately they have been using acetyl L-carnitine to slow down the aging process in the brain, and they recommend a higher dose for people at risk for Alzheimer's disease.

The Linus Pauling Institute also uses alpha lipoic acids, which keep the liver healthy. When your liver health functions well, your emotions are much better. All this is interrelated. Of course, we should not forget omega-3, our fish oil.

As you get older, you need to eat more of a plant-based diet because a plant-based diet will actually prevent small vessel disease. Small vessel disease is the problem that we have with aging. All the small blood vessels get clogged up with plaque. If you eat a plant-based diet, slowly you hopefully can actually decrease the clogging and improve nutrients for the brain cells. This is the approach that we use. Go on a plant-based diet, take omega-3, alpha lipoic acid, and acetyl L-carnitine.

DR. KONDROT: Some of the listeners may not be familiar with the homeopathic approach.

DR. LIM: I use homeopathic remedies for people who need help with concentration and learning or some older adults who don't really want to take any more drugs. I give them *cerebrum compositum*, which is very good if you take the correct dosage.

I usually give about six pills a day on alternate days. The pills are all taken under the tongue. It actually seems to help.

DR. KONDROT: Of course, the homeopathic approach is nontoxic and is actually a general stimulant.

DR. LIM: Remember, the most important thing is that your diet is the key. You need to go on a plant-based diet as you age. Nutritionally, the body prefers a plant-based diet. Of course, you can keep yourself healthy by volunteering or doing other things that keep your brain more vibrant. I would recommend the protocol that's proposed by the Linus Pauling Institute. Keep your brain cells healthy by using antioxidants and vitamin C. Use nutrients for the brain like fish oil and then, of course, the other things that our bodies don't make as much as we age. Your liver health is very important because your liver health controls your blood glucose. Once the glucose metabolism is better, your brain will be fueled better. To me, in aging, the most important thing is your brain. If the brain is aging too fast, it's not good.

The other part about aging is bone health. I always worry that as you get older, even for me, that mobility may be more limited. I tend to look at nutrition first and then the vitamins.

Vitamin D is very important in bone health. When women are menopausal, I try to tell them they have to rebalance their medicine. They can use botanicals like cohosh. I use a lot of evening primrose because I think it helps the mood, too. That's the way we approach it.

The biggest problems I see are in the big kids. In teenagers and people in their 20s and early 30s, we use the same approach as we use for adults. Thyroid health is very important. I always encourage people to make sure the thyroid is functioning optimally.

DR. KONDROT: One of the biggest problems that we see is obesity, not only in children but also in adults. I wonder if you could talk a little bit about your integrative approach in helping folks with obesity to get their health back.

DR. LIM: We see a lot of kids getting chunkier. The first thing I tell the parents is that I use the formula 95210. The nine is for nine hours of sleep. Five is five servings of fruits and vegetables. The two is not to use the computer quite so much, not more than two hours. One is one hour of exercise a day. Zero means everything they drink should be zero calories.

A lot of the time they're taking in many extra calories in their drinks. I know Gatorade is popular. Juices are very popular. I encourage parents to use more water. For the older kids, I think it's good to drink chamomile tea and even green tea.

The other thing we teach is that what you have on your plate should be 50% green. I always joke with the kids and say, "You know the color of money, which is green. Make sure 50% of your food is green, 25% is your protein, and 25% is the other."

We do see more and more Type 2 diabetes in children. We have to show them that, if they are really serious, it's 100% correctable by nutrition.

People also use medical food, which is intended for the dietary management of a disease that has distinctive nutritional needs that cannot be met by normal diet alone. Medical food is superior to regular food because it is metabolically balanced. These patients then combine a plant-based diet with medical food and good oils. The protocol is very efficient. We have people who have lost a lot of weight. We then have to teach them how to maintain. Insulin resistance is the most challenging because you have to really inspire them and make sure they sustain their effort.

DR. KONDROT: What about your approach with adults?

DR. LIM: Adults are the same. I may see adults who weigh 250 pounds. When they first come in, I do a baseline evaluation. I want to make sure their liver is healthy and they don't have gallstones. Then I tell them to go to a plant-based diet. We use the protocol from Metagenics called "FirstLine Therapy." We've been using it for many years, and it has been very successful.

We show them the ten classes of food they need to take. The majority of them are plant-based. We tell them, "If you really want to eat cashew nuts, you may be allowed to eat only eight a day and no more." The other thing is they need to learn is what makes a healthy snack. They're going to use things like cranberries, raisins, or veggies. The protocol from FirstLine Therapy is encouraging because they give you exactly the amount of caloric intake according to your weight.

DR. KONDROT: Dr. Ruth, I want you to talk a little bit about your use of hormonal replacement therapy, both in men and women.

DR. LIM: I do a lot of hormones for women. I'll talk about women first. The women actually start from a very young age. Some teenagers already have estrogen dominance syndrome. They don't have enough progesterone. Some of them have polycystic ovary syndrome (PCOS). I discourage them from using birth control pills, which is the allopathic option. I've been very successful using GUNA-PMS. Then, of course, I encourage them to go on a plant-based diet. I do use some homotoxicology drops, but the GUNA-PMS has been very successful, I would say. I had a couple of patients who had PCOS and ovarian cysts that were documented by ultrasound. Over time, the cysts become smaller, and actually, periods become more regular.

For the more mature women, we divide them into two groups. One of them is the premenopausal. They're going to go into menopause. They still have their period. Then there's the group that absolutely is already menopausal. Many times, they do not know what to do because of their symptoms. I encourage them to look at their nutrition first because I believe the Japanese are correct in recommending that they eat a lot of seaweed and a plant-based diet. I do give them options to see which way they want to go. I like to use oils, like evening primrose. I use botanical drops first, rather than the hormone cream. The botanical drops I use are GUNA-PMS or GUNA-FEM, and then, occasionally, I will prescribe GUNA-MALE, even for women. Women do need some testosterone. Otherwise, they always have palpitations and anxiety.

I do order saliva testing. When I look at the values, and, if they're really low and depleted, I will also use homeopathic creams. I use those, both the estrogen and progesterone, depending on the saliva testing results.

3. The entire hormonal system needs to be balanced before replacement therapy can be effective.

The other thing that is very important is that hormonal therapy cannot be successful if your whole axis is weak. I make sure the thyroid and adrenal glands are healthy. If they are not healthy, they will pull the other functions down.

In my experience, your adrenal health is probably the most important because the adrenal glands are the ones that are the generator of the energy. They rest upon the kidneys. They're small glands in the shape of a grape, but they control a lot of things like androgen production in both the male and female. If you have adrenal fatigue, I will have to address it. I will test cortisol levels with saliva testing and rebalance them from there. If they have a sluggish thyroid or hypothyroidism, we have to rebalance it. Hormonal therapy is more than just replacement.

The other thing I encourage folks to do is some meditation, if they can. Meditation is really good. It really fuels the whole endocrine system.

The next thing I tell these women is that they need to do things that make them ecstatically happy, do something that is good for their well-being. It could be art, listening to music, or a craft. All of those are very important for healing. You can use all these creams, but if the other parts of your life are not balanced, it's not really worth it.

I don't have a lot of experience with men, but I do use very good male urologists who can help me. I had a case recently with a man in his 70s. His wife, who complained that his mood was really not good, brought him in and, of course, there were other problems. I did encourage them to see the urologist.

Meanwhile, I found out from taking his history that he was very stressed. We started to repair his adrenals. We used adaptogens, and I looked at his thyroid, which fortunately was okay. I looked at his nutrition. He was very low in vitamin D, also.

DR. KONDROT: Could you share some advice, not only for adults, but also for children?

DR. LIM: This is what I learned since 1996 in my own journey. The key is to follow the model of the Linus Pauling Institute to reduce inflammation by using plant-based nutrition.

The way to reduce inflammation is to have really good gut health. The gastrointestinal system has to be very strong. If you have good gut health, you make enough serotonin and dopamine, so you don't really need to go on Prozac, Lexapro, Zoloft, and all that.

In order to have good gut health, nutrition is the key. Have a plant-based diet and eat for your blood type. Make sure you take probiotics. I use the 22 billion from Ortho, and I also use L-glutamine that repairs the lining of the gut.

These two things are very important as the basics. They will reduce the episodes of allergy. Asthma and eczema will improve. Actually, the other big thing I also talk a lot about is that you have to get rid of junk. You have to clear. The gut health and elimination is important. Make sure they eliminate well. I check their urine and make sure they don't have acidic urine and are drinking enough water to keep their body alkalized. That's really important.

Then besides the drainage, I also do immunomodulation, a technique that you can use to boost the immune system. Basically, I use a lot of adaptogens to boost the immune system. In the adult population, I use botanicals, including ashwaganda, ginseng, and rhodiola. In children, I use the gallium drops as I mentioned earlier. They seem to do very well.

....

RUTH TAN LIM, MD MD(H), FAAP FAAARAM
Dobson Integrated Medical Center
2058 S. Dobson Rd Suite 6
Mesa, AZ 85202
(480)820-4507

Michael D. Margolis, DDS

MESA, ARIZONA

Interviewed October 27, 2013

1. **You may have a genetic propensity toward mercury poisoning.**

2. **Don't do general detoxification until you have detoxified your mouth.**

3. **After a root canal, often the problem does not occur at the tooth but at an associated organ.**

DR. KONDROT: There is renewed interest in dental health and how our teeth are related to our general health. More people are becoming concerned about mercury amalgam and root canals and how they're adversely affecting their health. In my ophthalmology practice, I've come across many patients with chronic disease who have improved once they've seen an integrative dentist and had their amalgams removed.

Dr. Michael Margolis is an integrative or biological dentist in Arizona. He's also a member of the Arizona Homeopathic and Integrative Medical Association. His website is a resource for anyone who wants to learn more about how the teeth are connected to the rest of the body.

Please tell us a little bit about your background. Was there something that occurred in your training or practice that shifted your thinking toward biological dentistry?

DR. MARGOLIS: Like all dentists, I was trained to put in mercury, do root canals, and never really think about what I was doing because I was a tooth carpenter. I didn't even look at blood chemistries on patients to see how healthy they were. They were just supposed to be able to handle anything that the dentist did. It's quite amazing how well we were taught to be carpenters, but when it came down to the medicine part of treating a patient, my training seemed to be lacking the clinical skill set.

I did a lot of root canals and a tremendous amount of mercury fillings. Then one day about 19 or 20 years into practice, people began coming in and challenging my techniques. My reply was to say, "The American Dental Association says it's safe. They say it's fine, that nobody has ever had anything but an allergic reaction to mercury fillings; that root canals are totally safe; and that the tooth with the root canal still functions and is alive even though it's dead in the mouth."

Then two things changed the type of dentistry I wanted to practice. First, I placed a little mercury filling in a 12-year-old girl on her upper-left first premolar, which is Tooth # 12. Three weeks later, her left eye started to twitch. They took her to the family physician, who sent her to an optometrist, who sent her to an ophthalmologist, who eventually sent her to a neurologist.

The neurologist sat down and said, "Let's look at all the things that happened prior to this event." About three weeks before, she got nice, shiny, silver filling. The American Dental Association calls it silver. Fifty percent of that filling is mercury. Mercury is the most toxic metal that can be placed in a human being. It's more toxic than lead and arsenic.

He suggested that they come back and see me. The mother called me and explained what her daughter had been going through. I called the American Dental Association for help. I asked for the scientific department and got a secretary. I explained the situation and she said, "No, that could never happen!" But it had just happened to my patient.

When the daughter came in, we got her numb and I took that filling out in the wrong way. I didn't know that you had to put a rubber dam on the person and that they should have separate oxygen and a lot of water keeping the mercury vapors from being released. I also did not know that it was important to protect my assistant and me. When I took the filling out and placed in something called intermediate restorative material, a non-metal temporary filling, her eye quit twitching within 30 seconds. After that day, I never placed another mercury filling.

DR. KONDROT: That story is really amazing. The thing that really disturbs me is why is the American Dental Association still supporting mercury.

DR. MARGOLIS: The answer is politics and economics. The last organization to own the patent and the rights to mercury fillings happens to be in Chicago: the American Dental Association. If they were to admit that mercury could be the cause of many degenerative diseases, there would be liability. In 2013, the International Mercury Treaty was signed by 42 nations to phase out mercury, including mercury amalgam fillings, in the world.

DR. KONDROT: Did the United States did sign that document?

DR. MARGOLIS: We were part of it. Charlie Brown of Consumers for Dental Choice participated and it did go through the government, so there will be a phase out. They signed the treaty in Minamata, Japan, where they had experienced mercury poisoning of their population from industrial waste.

DR. KONDROT: We're very fortunate to have integrative dentists like you who are aware of this problem. Please go into a little bit more detail about why the mercury amalgam is dangerous. A lot of people rationalize, "It's not all mercury. It's mixed. It's solid, not a liquid. So what if a little bit leaches out into the mouth?"

1. You may have a genetic propensity toward mercury poisoning.

DR. MARGOLIS: The problem is that mercury is a neurotoxin and it attacks the arms of the nerve fibers and breaks those down. You don't need a lot of mercury to do this. There is a genetic propensity toward mercury poisoning in the 19th chromosome, where we have apolipo-

protein structure, or APOE. The APOE has two proteins. Two could be cysteine, two could be arginine, or it could be a combination of cysteine and arginine. If you're lucky to be an APOE2 in which you have two cysteines, you could drink mercury and you'll pee it out of your body. If you have a combination of cysteine and arginine, you have a 67% chance of eliminating the mercury. If you're the APOE4, you're in trouble. You are going to have Alzheimer's, Parkinson's or autism. People still say, about these neurological conditions, "We don't know what causes this," but we've known this for years.

DR. KONDROT: That makes sense because certain individuals can have a mouthful of mercury amalgams and they don't have any problems, yet that young girl you talked about had that reaction. The question I have is what percentage of the population has this APOE4 defect?

DR. MARGOLIS: APOE 3 is about 67% our population, when a person has one arginine and one cysteine. I would estimate that 12% to 15% would be an APOE 4, which is a very large number of people.

DR. KONDROT: Even if you don't have that genetic defect, chances are that the mercury is going to have a toxic effect on your body if you live long enough.

DR. MARGOLIS: It can cross the blood-brain barrier and cause neurological damage because mercury has an affinity for fat tissues. Your brain consists of fat, so mercury is extremely poisonous. A pregnant woman could be fine, but the developing fetus might inherit one cysteine from the mother and another cysteine from the father and could be poisoned by the mercury fillings in the mother's mouth! The problem is that some people don't get affected by it. With others, their lives are ruined as a result of it.

DR. KONDROT: Mike, please talk a little bit about that test to determine if you're in the group of people who have are most susceptible to mercury toxicity and where folks can request that test. This test is so important if you're having strange neurological problems or poor health and you don't know what in the world is causing it.

DR. MARGOLIS: It's easy to do if you go to a biological dentist or some alternative physicians who can order the test. Dental DNA of Colorado Springs has a simple saliva test. We can take samples and send it to the lab and within a week or so get the results back. That will tell you if you're at risk of toxicity or poisoning from mercury.

The other test that we run routinely for our patients is called the Clifford Materials Reactivity Test. This is a blood antigen test. You do not need to fast for it. We do it Monday through Thursday in our office. We have kits that are already made with directions. You can either get your blood drawn here by one of the doctors or you can go to a lab. The sample is spun, and then your plasma is sent to Colorado Springs where the results will tell you if you're reactive to over 10,000 dental materials used in dental offices in the United States today. It is an amazing, easy test. That one costs approximately $300, plus whatever the doctor or lab charges you to draw your blood.

It has been very accurate, but I always have to tell patients that when you get a blood reactivity test, it is a place in time. It may say that you're not reactive to something. Then you get a new material introduced to your body and three to five weeks later, you might be reactive to those materials.

We have referred our patients to homeopaths and naturopathic physicians who do allergy eliminations techniques. If they are reactive, sometimes that allergy can be reversed by another physician.

DR. KONDROT: I see patients whom I know have mercury amalgams, and they have eye disease or some other chronic problems. I'm sure some people are thinking, "My goodness! I've got mercury amalgams. When do I need to get them removed?" Do you take the position that everyone should get them removed, or is there a certain indication when you really have to look at getting them removed?

DR. MARGOLIS: I think that every mercury filling needs to be removed. Last week, I had a patient in who told me that her dentist said it was more dangerous to remove the mercury fillings than to leave them alone. That is because her dentist doesn't know how to remove the mercury fillings properly.

You want to go to a dentist who has been trained by the International Academy of Biological Dentistry and Medicine standard of practice and the International Academy of Oral Medical Toxicology standard of practice. We make sure that the patient is appropriately draped. We make sure that you're using a rubber dam, high suction, copious amounts of water, and a special fan that cleans the air around the patient. It is imperative that the patient has a separate supply of oxygen.

We also add charcoal to the protocol. Some doctors will do IV vitamin C. Do not take oral vitamin C because that breaks down in your liver and causes the anesthetic not to last in your body, and then it starts to hurt. An IV vitamin C is not a bad thing to have while you're having the mercury removed. The charcoal is a scavenger. It allows your body to get some of the bad stuff out that might get into your system while this is being done. The whole thing is a very systematic approach to doing it well.

If the doctor says, "Open your mouth. I'm going to take the mercury fillings out," get out of that chair as fast as you can. You're in the wrong place. The doctor doesn't know how to appropriately remove the toxins in your body.

DR. KONDROT: Unfortunately, I'm one of those doctors who usually advises patients that, if they're not having trouble, not to get the mercury amalgams taken out. I always felt that if the mercury was locked in that cavity and not causing any symptoms, it could cause more trouble if you get it removed.

After listening to you, I think that I'm going to be a little bit more aggressive because I believe the position you're taking. If it's not causing problems now, it probably will in the future.

DR. MARGOLIS: What problems are we talking about? I see so many patients with digestive problems, arthritis, fibromyalgia, and chronic fatigue; things that we can't explain very well.

2. Don't do general detoxification until you have detoxified your mouth.

Then we get these patients going into naturopaths and homeopaths who say, "We're going to detoxify you." They start a detox program with a mouth full of mercury. They're pulling the mercury out of the teeth into the body and giving them more toxins. My feeling is that the mercury in the mouth needs to be removed, and the patient needs to be nutritionally supported. As soon as that mercury and stuff is out of there, at that time you can go ahead and start detoxifying the person.

DR. KONDROT: What are you going to replace the mercury with?

DR. MARGOLIS: I use composite resins. They do contain Phenol A and that is not good for you. When they put the white filling material inside the tooth, the assistant takes a special infrared light at a particular frequency. It will set the material at 99.9% of hardness within 20 seconds.

I tell my staff to use the light for 30 seconds because doing it longer is not going to hurt it, but if you do it less, Phenol A could get released, and that is not healthy for the body.

DR. KONDROT: Dr. Mike, you have a story to share with us about how you were introduced to the dangers of root canals.

DR. MARGOLIS: Yes, I do. I personally experienced the dangers of root canals. I was taking a class in Minnesota on temporomandibular joint dysfunction (TMJ) and how to treat it. I went out to dinner with some friends that night, and we got rear ended by a tow truck going 45 miles an hour while I was doing zero. I became an instant TMJ patient. I had the misfortune of already having a root canal on my upper right first molar, Tooth #3.

In five days, my neck went from 17.5 inches to 24 inches around; I had kidney stones twice in the next two months; and if I ate any food, I would get tremendously bad gas and an upset stomach. It was the worst experience of my life. I was misdiagnosed with thyroid cancer and was told I would have to have my thyroid out. The biopsy report showed the thyroid was

totally normal, but I became a diabetic as a result of the misdiagnosis.

If you go to my website, www.mydentistaz.com, and go to the bottom of the page and look at the chart, "Meridian Tooth Chart." Look at Tooth #3. All the health problems I experienced were there. I had kidney stones twice that summer, and that's on the chart. It shows thyroid and pituitary glands, kidneys, stomach, and pancreas, which turned out to be all of my symptoms after the car accident and that root canal. I had the root canal taken out and all of these other symptoms went away except I became a diabetic. Root canals have some very dangerous implications in the body.

I use two laboratories, Fry Laboratories of Scottsdale, Arizona, and Dental DNA in Colorado Springs, Colorado, to do DNA testing. What we are finding are some very nasty viruses, bacteria, fungus, and protozoa in these biopsies. They're found inside a root canal tooth, which is a dead organ. How many dead organs do you want in your body?

Dr. Steinman at Loma Linda University did a study that demonstrated the physiology of these pathological situations. He injected radioactive dye into the dentinal tubules that make up the inner part of the tooth. Outside the pulp and inside the root, these are only 30 microns in diameter.

He was able to show, by placing a specially prepared dye small enough to get into dentinal tubules of a tooth in a dog and a cat, that the blood and lymphatics came through the pulp canal up throughout the entire dentinal tubule system, bathing that tooth with life, oxygen, and food. Then it would go out through the periodontal ligament into the interstitial space, the bone around the teeth. That's how the waste got out, along with the lymphatics in the return of the blood.

When you do a root canal, you remove all of those structures and you hollow out the tooth so it no longer gets nutrition. It no longer has the natural pathways to remove the waste; therefore, the tooth is dead. It can't get any food into the proteins that are inside the tooth any longer. The amino acids and proteins will decompose.

Since the tooth is sitting in the periodontal ligament, which is the cushion that holds the tooth between the bone and the tooth, it serves four different functions:

First, it holds the tooth to the jawbone.

Second, it acts like a cushion when you bite down. It also acts as a plunger when you release your bite; the tooth moves up in the tooth socket. This action pulls the liquid from the canal and pulp through dentinal tubules out of the tooth into the periodontal ligament and bone around it.

Third, it gives you feeling without pain.

Fourth, it prevents bone growth. All ligaments hold bone to bone. If the ligament is not properly removed from the tooth socket, your brain will think the tooth is still present and the site does not heal correctly.

DR. KONDROT: Three is enough to convince me that it is a serious problem when you have a root canal. When somebody comes in with a history of mercury amalgams or a root canal, the first thing I do is refer to your meridian chart. I want to know what's going on with that tooth and what meridian and organ it is connected to. Being an eye doctor, I'm interested in the liver and the kidneys, but primarily the liver meridian. It's a great chart and a great educational tool.

I'm still a little confused. I understand that there are two issues. The first is the danger of an infection after a root canal, and the other is this whole idea of the energetic meridian. I wonder if you could talk a little bit more about both of those. There is also the idea that when you have a root canal you're opening up these channels to an infection. No matter how good the dentist or dental surgeon is, even though they inject antibiotics and sterilizing agents, it's not going to clean that root canal.

DR. MARGOLIS: Basically what happens is the back teeth have three and a half miles of dentinal tubules filled with protein or amino acids. When the amino acids can't get oxygen and food, they decompose. This situation attracts various forms of bacteria, viruses, protozoa, and fungus looking for a food supply. There's nothing that stops them from going into the dead tooth. When the tooth was alive it had a hydrostatic pressure pushing out from within. That pressure is no longer there.

The inside of the tooth decomposes and the bacteria or these organisms are going to find their way in. You usually get pus, swelling, and heat in a normal infection. The root canal is a low-level, subclinical, toxic situation, but when it boils up, you've got pain, abscess, and you're hurting really bad.

3. After a root canal, often the problem does not occur at the tooth but at an associated organ.

The problem here is that it's subclinical. The problem does not usually occur at the tooth. It goes to the focal infection theory. Along the meridian that connects with that tooth is an organ at a distance away from the tooth, which can become ill, dysfunctional, sick, or infected.

DR. KONDROT: It's like in your case where you had the diabetes, problems with your pancreas, TMJ, and neck issues. Does everybody with a root canal have an infection?

DR. MARGOLIS: I would say anybody who has had a root canal for over 18 to 24 months will have a toxic situation with that tooth because of the decomposition of the proteins inside the dentinal tubules. This is even in the endodontic literature.

I know a number of dentists who say if you treat the tooth with ozone you're going to clean it out. I question if that is

possible since the natural mechanisms to keep the tooth "toxin free" are destroyed. Here is the problem: Within 18 to 24 months after the procedure, you're going to have bacteria buildup in the dentinal tubules because your immune system can't get inside the tooth and it's empty. That's where your bacteria, viruses, protozoa, and fungi are going to collect. I've talked to a number of alternative physicians who tell me that 98% of their women patients who have breast cancer and other cancers also have a root canal in their mouth.

DR. KONDROT: It is really alarming to think that a root canal can cause this much damage to your body.

DR. MARGOLIS: Unless a physician is trained to look, they're never going to make the connection between disease in the body with root canals, past extraction sites, or materials used in a patient's teeth since there is no pain. People think that unless you have pain in the mouth you're not having any problem. That's just wrong.

DR. KONDROT: In my practice, any time I see a strange diagnosis or organ problem I don't understand, I always ask the patient if they have had a root canal, and then I check with your meridian tooth chart to see if there's a correlation.

I wonder if you could illustrate this problem with some true-life cases.

DR. MARGOLIS: The first one I'd like to talk about is a 54-year-old Caucasian male. His chief complaint was that he had severe, painful arthritis of his right hand. This affected everything he did because he was a right-handed person. He wrote with his right hand and had difficulty writing because of such pain. It started three years before he was referred to me. He had seen 24 physicians, most of them specializing in the treatment of arthritis. He had been placed on multiple drugs, which he eventually discontinued because of their side effects.

He had had two root canals and one titanium implant. He had all four of his wisdom teeth extracted. He had four amalgams in his upper back molars on the right, one on the upper left and one on the lower right, and five metal-base crowns.

We haven't discussed the effect that many porcelain crowns have. They have a metal base underneath them with five or six different metals. This creates a galvanic charge throughout the whole mouth, which means that you've got a battery in your mouth.

His two root canals were his upper right canine and his lower second left molar. He had five missing teeth, including the four wisdom teeth and the one lower molar that had a root canal in it.

His gums looked pretty darn good. His X-rays showed that there were small abscesses at the base of each one of his root canals and that the titanium implant had not integrated very well into his bone.

I use a machine that's called a CAVITAT™, which is an ultrasonic imaging machine that was FDA approved. I was part of the research team that did the research on this machine that showed that it was 99.6% accurate with histological (microscopic) reports. With something called affinity-labeling technology, which no longer exists, it told me how toxic the areas were and helped me make a plan.

We went in and took out the mercury fillings, cleaned everything up, and used a Clifford test to see what materials to replace them with. I removed the root canal in the upper front. We cleaned his third molar areas on the right, which was his upper right and lower right Molars 1 and 32, and we removed (extracted) the titanium implant.

When this gentleman originally came in, and I tried to shake his hand, he pulled it away, explaining that he had so much pain that if anybody touched his hand he would be on the floor. He returned 15 days after dental surgery, put his hand out, and shook my hand. For the first time, he was brave enough to do that. He had no pain or ill effects. He told me he was 90% to 95% better. To me that was a miracle. I couldn't believe all that had occurred, and now he lives a normal, wonderful life. He's doing very well. He has no symptoms, and his wife is the happiest woman in the world.

DR. KONDROT: What do you think was the connection? Were the toxins in his mouth causing the arthritis or was it the meridian problem with the tooth?

DR. MARGOLIS: I think it was a combination of everything. As biological dentists, we are removing each layer like an onion, and each layer has an effect. I think that the mercury fillings and the metal-based crowns that he had in his mouth created a battery which lowered the gentleman's immune system. He also had leaky gut syndrome and gastrointestinal problems.

We just had to literally take our time and go through and take each layer off. We started with the metals and got those out. He felt a little better, but his hand did not improve. Not until we removed the root canal, cleaned out the past extraction sites, and took out the titanium implant on that side did his health improve. That was the final key. It was a combination of lowering the toxic load on his immune and neurological systems.

DR. KONDROT: Let's say this individual went through a very aggressive detox program with oral detoxification agents or IV chelation. Do you think it would have been successful?

DR. MARGOLIS: This is why I love this one homeopathic MD who sends me these patients before he gets started. He recognizes the importance of my work before he begins detoxifying his patients.

DR. KONDROT: I think this is a common mistake that a lot of integrative and

alternative doctors make. They'll see somebody who's toxic and begin IV therapies without looking at the underlying cause that could be in the mouth.

If you're having toxic symptoms, getting tons of IVs, and taking detoxification agents on your own without getting better, you've got to look in the mirror and look at your mouth. Do you have anything going on there that may need to be addressed first?

....

MICHAEL D. MARGOLIS, DDS, DOCTOR OF INTEGRATIVE MEDICINE
My Dentist
2045 So. Vineyard, #153
Mesa, AZ 85210
(480)833-2232
mydentistaz.com
info@mydentistaz.com

Dorothy Merritt, MD

HOUSTON, TEXAS

Interviewed November 17, 2013

1. One of the most important environmental problems is the amount of lead people who were born before the 1980s have been exposed to.

2. Lead is the number one cardiac risk; yet, people don't even know it. They obsess about cholesterol instead.

3. One statin is not equal to another statin. There's a big difference among them

DR. KONDROT: We have another very exciting guest, Dr. Dorothy Merritt from Houston, Texas. I wonder if you could share with us a little bit about your medical education and how you shifted more toward alternative treatments and what you're doing now. Then we can learn more about your practice and the innovative things that you're doing.

DR. MERRITT: I went to University Of Kansas Medical School and did my specialty training in Internal Medicine at Baylor College of Medicine in Houston, Texas, and I am Board Certified in Internal Medicine. I also became board certified in Hospice and Palliative Care Medicine when it first became a specialty in 2000. My most important post grad training was a six-month course in Environmental Medicine taught at the Southwest College of Naturopathic Medicine by Dr. Walter Crinnion, ND, and it changed my life and my medical practice more than anything I have ever done.

I never thought of myself as "alternative," but that's what people call you if you do things 10 to 15 years ahead of the rest. Even when I was a medical student in Kansas, I was traveling all over Kansas in a plane with my cardiology preceptor who was providing angioplasty, then a new treatment for coronary blockage. When I got to Baylor and the trials on this treatment were just starting, they were aghast that I had been doing it for years. I guess that was the beginning of my "alternative" career in medicine.

DR. KONDROT: Right now, I think that most traditional Western doctors would think that your practice is kind of strange. You're doing chelation, microcurrent treatment, thermography, and electrodermal testing, as well as a lot of other things in addition to daily care of adult patients. You have to admit that these things are just not accepted by mainstream medicine.

DR. MERRITT: That's right, and they won't be for another five to fifteen years, but there are always a few people who are looking ahead, and there are a few people back there dragging their feet. Ninety-nine percent of the people are in the middle trying to keep the status quo, and I'm just in the one or two percent that like to get out there and stir things up, and it's okay. I learned early on that it was very cost effective to practice preventive medicine in the days when they rewarded you for spending less money and having a higher quality of care. I came out on top, to the puzzlement of many of my peers, who no doubt were concerned with my approach.

Some of my peers thought I had become a total quack when I started doing chelation, and I even had the "honor" of having a complaint issued to the medical board by the head "quackbuster" in the United States. I won, but it took eight months of pure stress and $30,000 in legal fees. Now that there are two publications that have come out of the Trial to Assess Chelation Therapy (TACT) trial (I was one of a hundred principal investigators), which show huge improvements over "standard of care" especially in diabetics, I feel vindicated. However, despite the positive results, the medical "status quo" is still saying we have to do more studies before they can recommend chelation universally.

DR. KONDROT: I know you emphasize detoxification and chelation in your practice to get rid of heavy metals, especially lead. I wonder if you could explain why that is so important. Why should people be concerned about their lead levels and why should we get rid of lead?

1. One of the most important environmental problems is the amount of lead people who were born before the 1980s have been exposed to.

DR. MERRITT: There are several basic principles I use to get to the bottom of why my patients have medical conditions: genetics and environmental and nutrition deficiencies. One of the most important environmental problems is the amount of lead people who were born before the 1980s have been exposed to. From the early 1900s until mid-1970s, we poured so much lead into the environment that when they tried to test rocks to see how old the earth was, they thought that the earth was twice as old as it was, but it was due to the lead contamination on the rocks they were testing. In the 1950s and '60s, it wasn't unusual to have a blood lead level of 20 to 30 micrograms/dl, and now the average in the U.S. is about 1-2 micrograms/dl. Unfortunately it's still in our bones.

In 1979, a couple of years after they took it out of fuel, and subsequently paint, the lead levels in the United States dramatically dropped, but, unfortunately, 90% of it is still in your bones, and it comes out as you get older at a rate ten times "normal" aging and higher in ill patients.

2. Lead is the number one cardiac risk; yet, people don't even know it.

They obsess about cholesterol instead, which is minor compared to lead. Most doctors don't recognize lead toxicity, even though it's been published in all the top journals as a major cause of vascular, neurological, renal, and other degenerative diseases. Five years ago, *Circulation*, the American Heart Association journal, published an editorial entitled "Low Level Environmental Lead Silent Killer in US." Most of my cardiology friends saw the article but shrugged and said

we just don't have a treatment. When I mentioned EDTA Chelation, they just laughed.

There really is something you can do to get the lead out: EDTA chelation has been FDA approved for lead removal since the 1950s. Get tested; get treated; get the lead out! I have developed a program to document and treat people for lead toxicity with the new lower values, and I have had some luck with certain insurance companies cooperating with payment.

DR. KONDROT: You made an interesting comment. You said that as we get older, lead contained in the bone is released. I wonder if you could explain that in more detail.

DR. MERRITT: Ninety percent of all the lead you ever were exposed to, particularly back in the days prior to removal from gas and paint, has been calcified into your bones. That's fine until you're in your 40s, and then it starts coming out four to ten times faster than it did when you were younger just because of aging and hormones. It is even worse if you are sick. All of a sudden you're your own source of lead toxicity. You don't have to worry about it being in the paint or gas or anything anymore because you are your own source.

The CDC reduced the toxicity level to 5 micrograms for children in 2012. We used to think 20 to 40 micrograms/dl was normal but now we know that any amount of lead is toxic. There is no known level of lead that isn't toxic, and right now we've got a couple generations to go until we get all of this lead out of our bones. We need to chelate people because lead causes so many medical problems.

DR. KONDROT: I have two questions for you. How can people get their lead levels tested? The second question is what percent of the population do you feel has some toxic level of lead that needs to be treated?

DR. MERRITT: An article was published in *Circulation* in 2006 that reported that 38% of people in the United States have a lead level over two, and it was responsible for 180% to 250% of the increased death rate from heart disease. A similar article was published in 2009 in *Circulation* showing that if bone levels were measured, there was proof that the upper third of the population had 800% to 900% increased death rate from cardiovascular causes. That is the group we should be concentrating on because they are at tremendous risk. This is approximately two to three times more important than diabetes, smoking, and cholesterol as a health risk.

Right now in the United States, we can measure bone and blood lead levels with a simple, cheap blood test. When your doctor does your yearly tests, ask for a blood lead level. Even if you have to pay for it, it is very cheap. The results will say that up to 20 is okay because that is the

old OSHA level, and it's woefully out of date. The level that is okay is zero.

The other way to find out how much lead is in your tissue and indirectly in your bone is to do a chelation challenge test. That involves taking an IV dose of EDTA, which is an amino acid that binds lead, and we measure your urine for anywhere from six to twenty-four hours afterward. If a lot of lead comes out with the chelator, then you have a level of lead that's putting you at risk for illness including vascular disease.

The blood lead level just tells you what you've been exposed to over the last two to three months, and half of that value is from your bones; the other half is from outside exposure. The chelatable lead that comes out in your urine on a challenge test tells you how much you're at risk for over the long period. We do both of those, but we start with the blood lead level.

DR. KONDROT: Which test do you feel is more valuable? Do you think that both tests are required, or do you think that folks can choose one test?

DR. MERRITT: It depends. When you live in Galveston County, there's a lot of current as well as old exposure to lead. We have a lot of historical homes and we're one of the centers for lead toxicity. I think a blood lead level is where you start, but that doesn't mean everything, because if you're 40 and you have a whole lot of lead in your bones, it's not going to show up on your blood test. It's only going to show up on a challenge test. They are developing a technology that measures lead in the bones. It's just not commercially available yet.

DR. KONDROT: How about hair analysis? Does that have any value in evaluating lead toxicity?

DR. MERRITT: I don't really think it has much value for lead. It may have more value for things like arsenic and mercury.

DR. KONDROT: Dr. Merritt, before we discuss treatment, I want you to discuss symptoms. Do people who have lead toxicity feel differently? Do they have any unusual symptoms? I know you mentioned the risk of heart disease and other cardiovascular problems, but what are some of the other symptoms that people may experience?

DR. MERRITT: We have a check sheet of the top symptoms and conditions associated with lead that we have our patients fill out. Chronic fatigue is a common symptom. Abdominal pain and pain in general is not uncommon. The first condition that shows up is probably hypertension. For people between the ages of 40 and 62 who develop hypertension, 90% or more are developing it because lead is leaking out of their bones. That has been proven. That was published in the *Journal of the American Medical Association* back in 2003.

The other symptoms are cerebrovascular and neurological. There can be neuropathy, brain fog, memory loss, and symptoms that are just typical in aging adults. Gastrointestinal symptoms are common and people who have a lot of abdominal pain and weight loss that nobody can figure out frequently have elevated lead levels.

There have been a lot of studies that the National Institutes of Health have conducted correlating various medical conditions to elevated lead levels. Chronic vascular disease, neurological degeneration and brain atrophy on MRIs, renal insufficiency, cataracts, how fast you walk, how weak your bones are, and the list goes on. Basically, the gamut runs from A to Z, so as a primary care physician, when I'm looking at a 40-year-old or older who has any symptoms at all, I'm looking for lead. I don't care if it's autoimmune or vascular. I'm looking for lead and nutritional deficiencies and environmental exposures.

DR. KONDROT: Once you determine that a person has lead in their body, what treatment options do you offer? What are the best treatments, how effective are they, and how long does it take to remove lead?

DR. MERRITT: It's very complicated because there are a lot of things to consider. You may have one person that has a lead level of ten and has no symptoms, and another person with a level of one may have a lot of symptoms. But the bottom line is that lead is a toxicant at any level. The degree of symptoms has to do with genetics. That is why one person may have severe problems and another virtually none.

But if you don't look for it, you can't treat it. I have found that the best way to treat elevated lead levels is to use the methylated B vitamins. I always use methylfolate and methyl B12, and there's an amino acid called N-Acetyl Cysteine (NAC) that helps to get the body's methylation cycle opened up and start to dump out things, including lead. It reverses a lot of the symptoms caused by lead.

Then there's DMSA that they use in children, which is an oral pharmaceutical that binds the lead. In my opinion, the best treatment in adults is IV calcium EDTA, which is a modified amino acid. It has been FDA approved since the '50s to get lead out. It is safe, if administered correctly. It is also the fastest way to get lead out of your body.

If you're having symptoms or if you have vascular disease, I suggest a chelation treatment twice a week, and once a week if you're older or have impaired kidneys. Get at least 30 to 40 treatments over the first year. After that, do maintenance once a month or every two months just to keep the levels down so as the bone releases lead, you are binding it up and deporting it so it cannot harm you.

DR. KONDROT: Please clarify exactly what a treatment is like. I'm assuming this is an intravenous treatment.

DR. MERRITT: Yes. I don't recommend the oral treatments for lead toxicity because only about 5% of the EDTA is absorbed in oral treatments. If you use a suppository or the oral tablets that have EDTA, you're not getting a whole lot of lead out, but it may be helping with other things, and people who use this method do report improvement in some symptoms. If you really need to get lead out, you need to take the IV treatments of EDTA or oral DMSA treatments because they get a lot of lead out every treatment.

The interesting thing is that people with vascular disease, particularly diabetics, also benefited from EDTA in the recent TACT trials sponsored by the government. EDTA (both sodium and calcium EDTA) probably works on blood vessels by removing metals which have been causing the vessel to contract, and also independently on the nitric oxide system, both actions which result in increased blood flow.

DR. KONDROT: You mentioned earlier about nitric oxide and the importance of helping methylation while you're doing chelation. I think this may be a little different approach than many doctors use. Can you explain the importance of this approach and what nitric oxide is?

DR. MERRITT: Absolutely. Sixty percent of people in the United States compared to 35% of people in the rest of the world have a mutation in their ability to process folic acid and B12. This cycle also involves production of nitric oxide, the substance that opens up arteries and causes increased blood flow. Lead slows this cycle down, so lead exposure plus this common mutation cause a lot of problems with blood flow. Ninety percent of my patients in the last six years have had these mutations and I give them all methylfolate and methyl B12,

DR. KONDROT: Please discuss in detail the results of the TACT study which was a national NIH study sponsored by the government that proved that chelation is very successful. Why was this study so significant and why did this shock the medical community?

DR. MERRITT: Back in about 2000, they convinced the NIH to do this $32 million study of chelation, with noted cardiovascular researcher Dr. Gervasio Lamas at the helm. Ninety-nine percent of scientists, including those who ran the trial, were saying, "It's not going to tell us anything but we'll do it, or we're never going to win the argument."

What they looked at was how chelation impacted major outcomes after a first heart attack, like a second heart attack, deaths, re-hospitalization, angina, congestive heart failure, and the need for bypass surgery. They looked only at people who had had previous heart attacks. It was supposed to include 3,000 people but it ended up being fewer because cardiologists were afraid to refer people because they thought it was

bogus, but they finally enrolled enough to get good data.

What they discovered was that diabetics with previous heart attack who had chelation had a 40% improved outcome over people who were just on standard of care treatment like beta blockers, aspirin, Plavix, ace inhibitors, and statins. Those with major left-sided heart attacks had a 36% improvement, and everyone else had an 18% improvement over standard of care.

Critics said it did not meet the goal of 25% improvement. But things like Plavix offer only about 13% improved outcome, yet we use them, and statins may be up to 20% improvement post heart attack. Here we have this EDTA treatment that, after 40 treatments, reduces recurrent heart attacks and death by 40% if you are diabetic, and 36% if you'd had a major left-sided heart attack. The second study published in 2013 was the total diabetic subset, and it showed that with EDTA and vitamins, the recurrent heart attacks were reduced 51% compared to current standard of care. Why aren't we marching everyone into chelation clinics and making sure they get treated?

At the American Heart Association meeting where they announced the first set of data, you should have seen the reactions of the major cardiology gurus. A few notable "experts," who have never chelated a patient in their lives, were jumping up and down and saying, "We can't explain how this happened. We can't do this therapy because we don't know why it works, and too many alternative people were involved." We were just sitting there thinking that this was a national, double blind, professionally controlled study that show a huge positive outcome, and these people were acting just like fools, accusing us of somehow cheating, so the study would look good. It was just absolutely amazing to see the vitriol and accusations that were generated by much "respected" doctors.

If you had a pharmaceutical drug that did anything close to what this generic EDTA did, Dr. Lamas would have been flown all over the United States in a private Learjet and would be giving presentations every day. It was very shameful and embarrassing to me as a scientist to see this disrespect. Everybody said, "It works, but how many people do you see doing it? We're going to have to do a bunch more double-blind studies to prove that it worked." It's just crazy. It worked and it's cheap. We should be offering it to people in the 40 to 50 age group, in my opinion, but especially to diabetics with vascular disease, where there is no doubt that it helps.

DR. KONDROT: Why is it that the traditional medical establishment came down so hard? It's pretty difficult to argue against statistics that were so strong.

DR. MERRITT: You explain that, and you'll explain politics in America to me because I surely don't understand. The study was good science; it was done correctly.

These people are just having emotional outbursts because for 50 years they thought chelation was bogus. They've called it crazy science and then all of a sudden it works, but it doesn't work the way they thought it worked, so therefore it's an inconvenient truth.

The old way of thinking was that chelation directly takes calcium plaque out of the arteries. That's not how it works. It works by removing lead and other things like copper and iron that cause arteries to contract, and it works directly on the nitric oxide pathways to increase circulation. It actually causes increased blood flow to an area. When you get increased blood flow, you clean up an area, so your body naturally reduces inflammation and remodels the area.

You get increased blood flow so people don't have heart attacks. They get more blood supply, and they don't go into congestive heart failure. It's very explainable from a scientific point of view, but most doctors aren't really scientists.

Here we have something that has been proven; we know it works, and people are acting crazy. Unlike most therapies, it's amazingly cost efficient. The thing is that it's not illegal to get chelation in the United States. Get it if you can. Find a practitioner near your area. Even if they don't know why it works, just do it because we know that it does work, particularly in diabetics. I just wonder how long it will take insurance companies to rebel and pay for it since it is so cost effective.

Chelation is probably the number one thing that I recommend to patients, in addition to giving them the methylated folic acid and methylated B12, and N-Acetyl Cysteine NAC. These two treatments work faster than anything I know to heal patients and get rid of unwanted symptoms and conditions. The longer-term treatment is going to end up being microcurrent, a therapy you introduced me to.

DR. KONDROT: Please give us your opinion on statins and what this new study or new guideline indicated.

DR. MERRITT: The one thing they came out with was that it doesn't matter about the cholesterol level. If you've got somebody who is a high cardiovascular risk, you can put the fire out. I don't care what their cholesterol is; statins are fire trucks. They put out the fire.

If you don't want fire in your body because of inflammation, because you're not eating right or doing all of the other right things, statins probably do save lives for high-risk patients who are noncompliant with other lifestyle changes because they reduce inflammation.

3. One statin is not equal to another statin. There's a big difference between them.

Pravastatin and Livalo, which is the latest non-generic one, are the only two that don't cause elevated sugar and diabetes. With Crestor, Lipitor, Simvastatin, and Lovastatin there are increases in sugar levels.

I have mixed emotions about the statins. I think that if you have vascular disease, and you haven't changed your lifestyle radically, like going to a vegan diet, eating high nitric oxide foods like greens, and exercising, then you better take statins because we do know that they work in vascular patients, but they have a lot of side effects.

There are a lot of medications on the market that lower cholesterol but unless they lower inflammation, they are probably not worth it. They lower cholesterol, but cholesterol isn't the thing we're looking at. We're looking at inflammation, not a number. I think it's a real mess and I don't know how it's going to end, but I do know chelation will lower inflammation, increase nitrous oxide, and increase the blood flow. If I had to choose, I would pick chelation every time.

DR. KONDROT: Does chelation have any effect on lowering cholesterol?

DR. MERRITT: Not EDTA itself, but if you take methylfolate and methyl B12, you lower your homocysteine, and so you lower your heart disease risk. I've never seen a study where EDTA by itself lowers cholesterol.

DR. KONDROT: You commented that chelation could reduce the inflammation.

DR. MERRITT: Absolutely. There are

published studies that show this very nicely.

DR. KONDROT: Another really fascinating aspect of your practice is electrical medicine.

DR. MERRITT: That's not such a foreign concept. We've done EKGs and EEGs for years and now some company has put together the ES Teck Body Scan. It is a diagnostic test that combines five or six different electrical measures all in one. It takes about eight minutes, and I get this gorgeous measurement of every part of a person's body from head to toe from a real time physiological point of view. It shows everything. I can take a person who is kind of vague or who has a whole bunch of symptoms and, in eight minutes, I can pretty much surmise what is causing them and what they need.

The other thing I'm getting later this year or early next year is an EKG that has a chip in it that measures blood flow in each of the four major coronary arteries. It can tell the difference between something that's 50% or less blocked, 50% to 80% blocked, or greater than 80% blocked. It's called a MCG, and it is made by Premier Health.

DR. KONDROT: I don't know if you can answer this question, but what is the science behind it? In my mind, the only way to find out blood flow is to do it in a basic procedure and look at the blood. How is current related to blood flow?

DR. MERRITT: It's because someone has come up with a smart chip, like your smartphone; it can calculate blood flow in each of the coronary arteries based on the eight-minute blood flow that it's getting. You don't even have to do it with exercise. They can do it during a sleep study, just resting, or in the ER.

All of those people who come into the ER with chest pain get $10,000 or $20,000 workups because they have chest pain, but if they have less than a 50% blockage in an artery, their chest pain is not due to any coronary action, so you can send them home. Some of the major hospitals in Houston are putting these in their ER because, even if they don't get reimbursed, they can prevent these $10,000 unnecessary workups.

DR. KONDROT: I just read that now there's an EKG iPhone 4S. You can actually take your own EKG.

DR. MERRITT: Yes. I just upgraded my iPhone. You can just sit there and put it on the patient and read the EKG.

DR. KONDROT: Another thing that I'm really excited about is that you are beginning to use microcurrent stimulation.

DR. MERRITT: Thank you very much for introducing me to that. I have the units that you use on your eye patients and the ten different protocols that you programmed for me. Eighty percent of the patients I have treated are on half the amount of pain medicine than they were before treatment. Fifty percent of their pain is gone. I really thank you for introducing me to that technology because I think it is absolutely the future.

I know that it will work on pain, and I know it works on my eye patients for rebuilding their retina, so I'm just wondering if it will rebuild the pancreas or a heart. There are just so many what-ifs. I think this is the new future.

DR. KONDROT: You have so much energy. Before the radio show you were talking to me about developing new programs or protocols for different parts of the body.

DR. MERRITT: I think the future of medicine will be like having a library and you reach up and grab your thyroid microcurrent device and wear it tonight. Then you reach up and grab your pancreatic one. If you're like the rest of us, you're just going to reach up there and grab the ones you need. I think that's going to be so cool.

DR. KONDROT: Dr. Merritt, I wonder if you can offer advice to people who are not satisfied with their health or who have some type of illness that's not responding to conventional treatment.

DR. MERRITT: It probably depends on their age. The first thing is to get some form of methylfolate and methyl B12 and possibly N-Acetyl Cysteine (NAC)

and start taking those along with eating a healthy, organic diet high in greens. If you buy organic you sometimes get 1,500 more times the minerals and nutrients that are in regular food. Just throw out the boxed food and buy one or two things a day that are organic. Quit drinking sweetened and carbonated beverages because they're the number-one cause of diabetes in the world. Don't smoke. If you smoke, stop as soon as you can. Get EDTA chelation once every month or two if you're 40 or older and walk at least 15 or 20 minutes daily. Even if you're in bad shape, start walking. It takes 10 minutes to produce nitrous oxide, so walk 15 to 20 minutes to start with. Many things that you can do for yourself can have a tremendous positive impact on your health. We did not cover it, but I want people to know that I do non-invasive Nexalin treatments, a new FDA cleared treatment for depression, insomnia and that information is at www.nexalinhouston.com.

....

DOROTHY MERRITT, MD
Mainland Primary Care Physicians,
6807 Emmett F. Lowry
Expressway Ste 103
Texas City, Texas 77591
(409)938-1770
www.mpcptexas.com – practice website
www.SWWellness.com – website for articles

Nicholas J. Meyer, D.D.S.

SCOTTSDALE, ARIZONA

Interviewed June 30, 2013

1. In 30 seconds, I can change someone's complete autonomic nervous system as a way to illustrate the importance of their bite and how it affects their whole body.

2. When a tooth has a root canal, it harbors anaerobic bacteria that give off endotoxins, and the toxins travel throughout the body.

3. Dentists are required to handle mercury-filling materials as toxic materials before they are placed in your mouth. Are they safe inside your mouth?

DR. KONDROT: I respect Nick Meyer for his work in integrative dentistry. Since I became friends with him and since I've become his patient, I've learned that dentistry has expanded. It's more than just taking care of teeth and filling cavities. There's an amazing connection between the tooth and the whole body. How did you get interested in integrative dentistry?

DR. MEYER: I became a dentist 34 years ago. I went to Loyola University in Chicago and graduated in 1979. I was a card carrying member of the American Dental Association for maybe the first eight or so years of my practice. I did what I thought to be the best thing at the time, which was prescribing fluoride and doing mercury fillings. I thought nothing about doing root canal treatments. Over the years, as I attended different kinds of programs within the world of alternative medicine, I learned that perhaps mercury fillings weren't the best idea for people's health. That got me thinking about why that would be when I was taught that everything about them was okay. It has been an interesting journey since.

I've come to find out that most of the different political camps and factions within the profession revolve around the moneyed interests so that the status quo can be kept the same. Additionally, I feel that the powers-that-be have a sense that if people can stay just sick enough, there's going to be a lot of work for this whole medical-industrial complex that we're all part of.

DR. KONDROT: With most of the doctors whom I have interviewed, there was one pivotal event in their lives. For myself, I got severe asthma. Traditional medicine couldn't help, and homeopathy cured me. Is there a particular personal incident or a patient who really helped you to shift your perspective and thinking?

DR. MEYER: There *was* a defining moment. It was when I was a young practitioner. My office manager had to leave her job. She went out to a clinic in Las Vegas where she was diagnosed with multiple sclerosis.

She came back with a large packet of information that had come out of Germany. It talked about teeth as being organs. That was a new concept to me. I always thought teeth were just teeth and that organs were inside our body, like our heart, lungs, and things like that.

She had a listing of all kinds of electrical readings on her teeth and indications of what she was supposed to use to restore her teeth, etc. This was really an eye-opening event for me. I hung on to that material probably for 15 years. It was kind of like seeds that were planted in fertile soil. They were very slow to grow. As my awareness deepened and I became broader in my scope of what it means for me to be a dentist, the whole thing started to come together in a big way.

DR. KONDROT: One thing that I find really interesting about your practice is you have gadgets, lasers, and electrodermal testing devices. You represent a trend that's taking place in all of dentistry, which is that you're looking more at the whole body. I know you had a sleep apnea clinic for a while. You also have a lot of interest in the bite. I wonder if you could talk a little bit about how important our bite is, what it represents for our health and how you evaluate that particular issue with patients.

DR. MEYER: Thanks for the compliment about the gadgets. They're indispensable tools for what I do in my practice. It's not so much the tools that drive my practice. It's the philosophy of the practice that drives my need for certain tools.

1. In 30 seconds, I can change someone's complete autonomic nervous system as a way to illustrate the importance of their bite and how it affects their whole body.

I became aware of the importance of the occlusion, or the bite, in the mid '80s. I had been in practice for about six years. I was introduced to how the muscles of the head and neck, not just the muscles around the mouth, which I deal with, and the tongue but the whole upper quarter, come to bear on what it is that I do in dentistry and, as a result, in healthcare. I can take somebody and in 30 seconds change their complete autonomic nervous system as a way to illustrate for them the importance of their bite and how it affects their whole body in balance, structure, and alignment.

I started watching people's eyes and facial structures change by doing nothing other than putting balance back into a system. I stopped looking at teeth as the object of my efforts. I looked at them as a means to an end, that end being balance. So many more things came into focus for me. It really rounded out my whole perception and perspective of what dentistry is for people and can do for their lives.

DR. KONDROT: Is it the bite that causes the imbalance in the autonomic nervous system, or is it the imbalance in the autonomic nervous system that affects the bite?

DR. MEYER: The curious thing about the bite is that it's the end result of a very dynamic system of having all the teeth come together. When it looks like it's right, most people would just say, "Your bite is good." However, that is often just a masked end point of a dysfunctional system. If there's an imbalance of the jaw joints left and/or right and an imbalance of the muscles of the jaws and shoulders, which can stem out of misaligned hips, for instance, then you're going to have a system that is torqued in some manner.

Pilots understand this idea really well. If you look at how an airplane goes through space, it has pitch, roll, and yaw axes. We use the same terminology in dentistry when we describe how the jaw and the teeth come together and have a really good three-point landing.

That doesn't happen for a lot of people. The consequences of that are great. We talk about the autonomic nervous system and which comes first, the chicken or the egg. I have found that it works both ways. What I mean by that is you can have a traumatic event, such as a motor vehicle accident, which sets up a glitch in the system. A system that had been right previous to the accident or whatever the trauma is can now be dysfunctional. The autonomic system is immediately impacted from the trauma. When something like that happens and there's shortening of a muscle which pulls the jaw off a little bit, the teeth which normally nested very well together all of a sudden are striking at a different angle and pitch and with a different amount of force on new surfaces that had not been designed to take that load. We see exaggerated wear facets on teeth. You'll find fracturing and shearing of the cusps off the side of the tooth. In extreme cases, there's complete fracture of the tooth clear through the root stock. That's a pretty significant event. It is probably at the far end of the spectrum of the things that we see, but very commonly we see sheared off or fractured cusps.

DR. KONDROT: That's really interesting. You can just look at somebody's teeth and immediately assess whether there's an imbalance in the bite.

DR. MEYER: Yes. Related to that conversation are problems to the airway. It has been discovered, with the benefits of three-dimensional X-rays that the problems that go on with somebody's airway, particularly when they sleep, play out in their teeth and mouth. The bones that form on the inside part of somebody's lower jaw are called tori. Sometimes these are massive. They form in large measure as a direct result of an excessive amount of pressure or force on the jaw when the teeth are brought together. That is manifest at night as a result of an airway impediment.

When a person is biting their teeth together hard, the constrictor muscles of the airway are opening to allow air to pass through. When the clench is released, the muscles relax and the airway starts to collapse. There's a dance that goes on

throughout the night.

Somebody may come in to my office and say, "Doc, I have a toothache." I will ask them when it started and go through the whole history. Then we may see that the nerve died in the tooth. It could be a virgin tooth, but because of a compressive injury to the tooth, it has been suffocated. It's no different than a heart attack, but the person is having a tooth attack, if you want to think of it that way.

When the pain occurs, a dentist will do one of two things. We'll take the nerve out of the tooth so the pain receptors go away, or we'll remove the tooth. That also gets rid of the pain receptors. Either way, the pain receptors are out of the picture.

This is a very interesting thing. If you end up taking the tooth out of a clenching person, you'll further upset the dynamics of the jaw because the teeth are going to be shifting. It's going to change the dynamic of how the jaw is working. They'll end up with some clicking or popping and, later on, osteoarthritis within the joint.

There's a phenomenal cascading effect of problems that can all come from any one of those things we're talking about. It's all mediated through the autonomic nervous system.

DR. KONDROT: It sounds to me like an amazingly delicate balance in the mouth. When all systems are functioning fine, it's a beautiful operation. It seems to me like there are many different mechanisms that can malposition teeth or cause a problem with the bite. You were talking about respiratory difficulties. Is this related to sleep apnea?

DR. MEYER: Yes, it is. Respiratory difficulties are on a spectrum. You don't have to have overt sleep apnea, which is diagnosable by a particular set of numbers that somebody has per a sleep test. I have sent a number of people in the practice for sleep tests. They'll come back saying, "I don't have sleep apnea." That's good, but they still have a problem. Because they're so keyed in on sleep apnea as the thing that they're looking for, they ignore the fact there are other problems. They say, "If I don't have the apnea, then I must be okay." That's wrong. Their numbers, which indicate their symptoms, are just not in the range that triggers the medical diagnosis of sleep apnea. A person can have upper airway resistance syndrome, for instance, still causing problems in breathing but not triggering what would be officially considered sleep apnea.

DR. KONDROT: Even though it's not official sleep apnea, what type of ill effects could this have on a person?

DR. MEYER: Here they are in order of what I see happening in my practice. The most common one is temporomandibular joint (TMJ) problems from muscle overload. Related to that is myofascial pain dysfunction (MPD) which is purely the muscle manifestation of the problem. You could end up causing a slipped disc in the jaw joint. Now, you're getting into

some orthopedic issues within the point. That can cause muscle locking. A lot of pain comes along with that.

I have seen sheared-off cusps of teeth or wholesale loss of the tooth structure in a vertical direction. You take the beautiful topography of a tooth and make it flat as a pancake. Sometimes the teeth look like little cow pies. They're so irregular in the way they look that they don't really resemble teeth anymore.

Because of the over-compression of the blood vessels as they come into the teeth, it's like kinking a garden hose. You cut off the flow of blood, as well as the lymph, and you end up with toothaches. A simple thing that we do to help people, although it isn't curative, is the placement of a bite guard. A bite guard can really help disengage the teeth to eliminate some of the negative pressure that's being put on the structures.

DR. KONDROT: Let's tackle a very controversial subject, root canals. Should they be avoided entirely? What are the dangers of root canals?

DR. MEYER: The thing about root canals is that a tooth with a root canal, or that is said to need a root canal, is a dead part of your body. If dealt with in any other area in orthopedic medicine, like a toe, finger, or leg with gangrene, it would be off in a heartbeat because it's known that we cannot retain dead issue.

In dentistry, we've found a way to trick the body. We mummify the tooth, and then we put a wig on it in the form of a crown. That's a way that we have to keep a tooth functioning as a member in the mouth. The question today is should we do a root canal when there are other modalities available such as dental implants? I'm a very big believer in having the function of the system remain intact.

Back in the day when we didn't have the techniques available that we have now, root canals offered a way to retain a root so that a mouth could continue to function reasonably. The negative part aside, it was a noble effort to try to keep the tooth so it could function. Function in the mouth is so sacred, in my opinion. That's what drives the early diagnosis and treatment planning of people so that we understand the function, dysfunction, and how we can get them better.

2. When a tooth has a root canal, it harbors anaerobic bacteria that give off endotoxins, and the toxins travel throughout the body.

With the root canal situation, something has caused the nerve and blood vessels within the tooth to die. That could be from blunt trauma, clenching on the tooth, a mercury filling that was in the tooth, or a doctor drilling a questionably healthy tooth. As a result, the tooth was not able to do anything but have the nerve in the tooth die. With the advent of dental implants, the question is should we keep a tooth that has a root canal or not?

DR. KONDROT: We need to explain how lengthy the root of the tooth is and how it extends into the body. It's not just a one-inch structure. Isn't that so? We're dealing with something that connects with many different areas of the body.

DR. MEYER: That's right. What you're referring to is the energetic relationship that the teeth have to all the other body parts. We know through acupuncture that everything is connected through these energetic meridians. The teeth are no different. They are part and parcel of the whole system. It's just that they're not readily recognized and discussed in that world of acupuncture.

For instance, a small incisor in the lower jaw has microscopic tubules that run from the inside part of the teeth where the nerve is to the outside part of the tooth, the ligament space that holds the tooth in. It has been calculated that if you were to put those little tubules end to end from that one little tooth, that would extend approximately 3.5 miles. It's huge. If you have that kind of circuitry in just one tooth, when the tooth dies, bacteria in the body will go into those little tubules, because there's no more flow in them, and take up residence.

Here's the problem. The bacteria go from the air breathing type — not very harmful bugs in our bodies — to air hating. These live in an anaerobic environment. When they do that, there's a conversion to this anaerobic state, and they start to excrete endotoxins. These toxins are very harmful to the body. They're neurotoxins. When a tooth has a root canal, the endotoxins disrupt the flow of energy in the tooth and, therefore, throughout the system. The tooth harbors anaerobic bacteria that give off endotoxins. The toxins go all over the body.

They also have a way of causing the body to be dumbed down. The immune system turns a blind eye to most of these toxins that are in the body. They go off the radar until a crisis happens within the system and then show up as a problem. We have the energetic component and the endotoxin component, which goes throughout the system.

Here's an interesting story. A cancer clinic in Switzerland did a survey of 50-100 women who had breast cancer. Virtually every one of them had a root canal on an upper first molar. That molar is on the systemic meridian which runs through the breast.

With the lifestyle choices that women make, including bras, there's stagnation of fluid. Then they have these energetic and toxin problems from a root canal, and they end up getting cancer.

DR. KONDROT: I know that more integrative doctors are looking at this issue with root canals. There are charts of corresponding meridians and organs that relate to each particular tooth. In my practice, if I find that there's a history of a root canal, I want to know which tooth the root canal was done on. Then I look at the corresponding meridians and

organ systems. The pathology that can correspond to this is surprising.

DR. MEYER: It's pretty amazing. I actually have that chart several places in my office. We give that chart out when people come in and have root canal treatments in their mouth. We discuss it with them while they are making their decision to remove the tooth or not.

DR. KONDROT: For the person who has a root canal, what advice would you give them? Would you advise them to get the root canal corrected, and how is it corrected?

DR. MEYER: The only way to create a cure with a root canal is to remove the tooth. Having said that, removing the tooth sets off a cascade of other issues. If you take the tooth out, then you're going to have bone loss around the area where the tooth was. You're going to need a replacement tooth. You'll have three options for the replacement tooth: a removable bridge, a fixed bridge, or a dental implant. Very often, those are not really good options for certain situations. I don't have a good blanket answer for the question you asked because it requires a unique, individual answer for each situation.

I mentioned that function is important in my way of looking at things. I want to be able to help assure somebody that they're going to be able to have really good function. For instance, although dentures are teeth in somebody's mouth, they're roughly only 40% as efficient as natural teeth. With dentures, your efficiency and ability to masticate your food and have proper digestion goes way down, not to mention other aspects of your quality of life.

DR. KONDROT: The bottom line is that you really need to be evaluated by a dentist who's knowledgeable about all these issues. I know that you belong to an integrative dental association. Maybe you can tell us how to get in touch with an integrative dentist.

DR. MEYER: The organization that I'm a past president of is the International Academy of Biological Dentistry and Medicine. Our website is www.IABDM. org. There is a directory that will help direct you to a doctor in your location.

We're a pretty small, unique group of doctors. It's not uncommon for people to travel from quite a distance and even from other countries to find one of us and take advantage of our particular skill set. Not all doctors are created equal, as you well know. That's certainly true in dentistry. There's such a different flavor of discipline within dentistry. Some people don't give any credence to the bite. Other people do. Other people think only of mercury fillings, which I know we're going to chat about next, and on and on it goes. It depends on what a person is looking for. Are they trying to have optimum health or just have some short-term problem solved?

DR. KONDROT: We also have to discuss one of the most controversial topics, the issue of mercury amalgams. Please give us your perspective?

3. The Environmental Protection Agency wants us to handle mercury-filling materials as a toxic material before it goes into your mouth. It seems to be okay once it's in your mouth.

DR. MEYER: It's very simple. Mercury is one of the most toxic substances known to man. I think it is the most toxic non-radioactive substance. It's curious that the Environmental Protection Agency wants us to handle mercury filling materials as a toxic material before it goes into your mouth. It seems to be okay once it's in your mouth. Then once it comes back out of your mouth, it has to be handled as a toxic material again. There seems to be a big disconnect on the official side of things at the governmental level that mercury is okay as long as it's in the human body. Once I understood that way back in the mid '80s, it never made sense to me again.

Today, we like to think that we're enlightened, but approximately 45% of the teeth that are filled have mercury-based fillings. That could be a small one or a large one. We used to make jokes about it when we were younger practitioners. A single fill was one mix and it would be a small filling, but sometimes you'd be mixing five different packages of material. You'd be recreating the whole tooth out of a gumball-sized piece of mercury that we'd be putting onto the tooth. Then that would be held in place by stainless steel pins that would be driven into the tooth like little lightning rods.

The thing about mercury that many people don't know is that it volatilizes. It comes out of the filling in a vapor form. You have to understand that where those fillings are only inches away from your brain. It has been amply demonstrated that mercury has retrograde axonal movement. That means the mercury from the tooth can go backward through the nerve up into the brain. That's very frightening.

A number of years ago when Dr. Boyd Haley was doing his research with Alzheimer's disease and mercury, he was able to replicate, in the laboratory, the same neurofibrillary tangles that are seen in an Alzheimer's brain with the application of mercury to a rat brain, which is a fairly close physiological model for humans. The problem with that is when it's combined with other metals that are commonly used in dentistry such as copper and tin, you have a synergistic effect of these different metals and you get more massive destruction.

These are the kinds of things we're involved in when we help people by safely removing the mercury from their teeth. We call ourselves a mercury-safe practice. We go through some very unique steps in safeguarding the individual whose mercury we're extracting from their mouth, as well as our own health.

It is a toxic material. It has to be treated carefully.

DR. KONDROT: What are some of the indications that someone is suffering from mercury toxicity?

DR. MEYER: The most common ones are brain fog, unexplained irritability, urinary problems, and chronic fatigue. We talk about mercury, but there's another facet to it which bears consideration. A battery functions because of two dissimilar metals in the presence of an electrolyte. You have that in your filling. You have five different metals that are in a filling in the presence of your saliva, which is an electrolyte. You have phosphorous, calcium, etc. It's a soup in a nice, beautiful, warm environment, so you create these little batteries.

That causes the brain to have a higher amount of energy being supplied to it than what's normal to the working of the body. You get magnitudes of more energy going back into the system. This can explain why some people have immediate changes in their health when their fillings are replaced. It's not so much from the mercury phenomenon, but from the electromagnetic field and electrical energies that are dissipated immediately upon removing the mercury filling from the mouth. It's a very complicated and interesting area of biophysics of the head and neck.

DR. KONDROT: Is there a way that people can be evaluated through a blood test or measurements for mercury in their system?

DR. MEYER: There are a handful of ways to assess mercury in the body. There are blood tests. The most reliable tests are special and unique, not the typical ones that are ordered by your doctor's office. They can be ordered by your doctor if they know what they are. These tests can find out what particular species or forms of mercury are floating around in your body. It's a fairly new blood test that has been developed in the last five years or so by a laboratory in Colorado.

Another way to test is through an electroacupuncture screening using resonance. Muscle testing is another way to help try to get a handle on this. The mercury challenge tests, which are common in some of the offices of your colleagues, don't really tell you about the total body burden of mercury; they just reveal that your body has mercury in it. It is useful as a gauge in the detoxification that is undergone with a naturopath, homeopath, or somebody who's helping you through that particular process, but there are more specific measurements.

The important thing for people to understand is that dental health is intrinsically related to their total health. If they are having problems that cannot be solved within conventional or even alternative medicine, they may want to consult a holistic dentist.

....

NICHOLAS J MEYER, DDS
Millennium Dental Associates
Scottsdale, Arizona
(888)948-0560
www.milldental.com

David P. Nebbeling, DO

LANSING, MICHIGAN

Interviewed September 15, 2013

1. I practice miracle medicine.

2. People do not have to live with pain and arthritis as long as their body possesses enough healing ability to heal itself.

3. I've developed a special protocol for those with emphysema or COPD.

DR. KONDROT: Dr. David Nebbeling is my personal physician. I certainly appreciate all the care he's given me over the years. Please tell us a little bit about your medical career, how you got interested in alternative medicine, and describe what a doctor of osteopathic medicine is, and how they're different from medical doctors.

DR. NEBBELING: I grew up in East Lansing, Michigan. After completing my undergraduate degree at Michigan State University, I attended Michigan State Uni-

versity College of Osteopathic Medicine (MSUCOM). MSUCOM is renowned for its teaching programs in Osteopathic Manual Therapy (OMT). I went far beyond the required classes in OMT each term and took classes in the evening, on weekends, during the summer, and even sat in on continuing medical education classes for licensed DOs. I did my hospital training in Davenport, Iowa. It was there I met Wilber Huls, DO, and it was his practice, the Blue Grass Clinic, that I took over when I finished my hospital training in 1987.

Dr. Huls and his father before him were famous for their skills in OMT. Dr. Hulls showed me how to inject ozone gas into joints to treat osteoarthritis. The treatment is now known as Prolozone. He also showed me how to compound hormones and use them to put rheumatoid arthritis into remission, a process known as Liefman's Balanced Hormone Therapy. Before retiring, Dr. Huls introduced me to various doctors and organizations that specialized in alternative medicine to help further my education.

Osteopathy was developed by Dr. Andrew Taylor Stills in 1874 as an alternative to the medical practices of his time. Dr. Stills gave us four principles as guides to the philosophy, which was meant to grow with time and the advancement of knowledge.

PRINCIPLE #1: God gave the *body the ability to heal itself.*

PRINCIPLE #2: *Unity of the Body* - we are made up of a series of systems that are interdependent and interrelated, and we are made up of mind, body, and spirit. Osteopathy coined the term "holistic medicine" around 1900.

PRINCIPLE #3: *The reciprocal principle -* structure affects function, and function affects structure.

PRINCIPLE #4: *The rule of the artery is supreme.* Where we have good blood flow and uninterrupted nerve flow, you will find health and healing.

Dr. Stills also taught the laying of hands on the patient and the use of palpation for diagnosis and treatment. We call this part of osteopathy, Osteopathic Manual Therapy (OMT).

DR. KONDROT: I think those four principles are really interesting. If I had known this about osteopathic medicine, I would have probably pursued it instead of my traditional medical training. How do you actually assess a patient?

DR. NEBBELING: I'll use a patient with a poor functioning thyroid gland as an example. A traditional MD would perform one or two lab tests to determine if the patient has a thyroid problem and should be referred to a specialist. An osteopath would first examine the patient with his eyes and hands, looking for signs of health or disruption of health in the patient's hair, eyes, tongue, throat, skin, in the nervous system, and in the body temperature. The osteopath will ask a series of questions covering the systems of the body. The osteopath will also look at lab tests, but he or she will not take the traditional narrow view of looking at one or two tests for a specific number that supposedly signifies a particular disease. An osteopath will look at thyroid lab values as part of the spectrum of thyroid health and integrate that with other information he has gathered on all the other systems of the body. Finally, treatment options may include supplements with iodine and herbs to help detoxify the glands and improve the functioning of metabolic enzymes. Treatment of a thyroid dysfunction would also include testing for heavy metals and treating accordingly. If medicine were necessary, the osteopath would consider natural extracts of thyroid hormones or bioidentical thyroid hormones.

DR. KONDROT: Was there was a turning point in your career or did you start out looking at the holistic approach to healthcare?

DR. NEBBELING: I can say three events greatly affected how I approach medical practice today. The first occurred during high school. I wrestled heavyweight and had multiple low back sprains as a result of many hours of practice. One day when I was 16, I experienced low back pain that lasted over two weeks. My parents took me to one of the most famous orthopedic clinics in the 1970s for an examination. I was told I had six lumbar vertebrae in my low back, while most people have five. Further, I was told I had a weak low back, and I should never lift over 50 pounds if I wanted to avoid back pain. As an active 16-year-old who wanted to wrestle and lift weights, I could not accept this restriction. I started to look for an alternative way to prevent my back pain.

The second event occurred when I was a pre-medical student. I read a book by George Northup, DO, called *Osteopathic Medicine: An American Reformation*. The short book spelled out the osteopathic philosophy. These principles resonated with me, and from then on, I knew I wanted to be an osteopath and practice holistic medicine.

The third event occurred during my last year of medical school. My 15-month-old son, Caleb, was diagnosed with neuroblastoma. It was one of the most common cancers for a child to be born with — one out of 27 — but most children's healthy immune systems quickly destroy the cancer cell, so the actual number of children who develop tumors is about nine per million.

My son underwent chemo and radiation, which unfortunately were unsuccessful. During this ordeal, I knew in my heart that the way to fight cancer was to restore the body to health, not poison cancer cells and the immune system. I didn't know how to do that back then or where to take my son for that kind of help, but I started learning about detoxification, nutrition, homeopathy, and even inventive ways to use prescription medicine to restore the body to health. There had to be another way. How do we build the immune system? How do we work with that? That made me start looking for a different solution.

DR. KONDROT: You had the motivation and zeal to look at medicine from a holistic approach right from the beginning. Many of us who go into medicine are indoctrinated early on. That knowledge or that desire to truly help people look for the underlying causes is suppressed. It has to be developed later on because of frustrating personal experiences or finding out that you're really not helping people.

Could you tell us a little about your approach to the patient who comes to you with the problem and your methods of evaluation, your protocols, and your techniques?

DR. NEBBELING: The main focus of my practice for the past 25 years has been musculoskeletal medicine. I have very developed skills in palpitation, OMT, and employ many modalities and alternative techniques to help patients recover from pain in any joint or limb in the human body. Most common is knee pain followed closely by low back pain. I have very successfully treated head pain, thumb pain, foot and ankle pain, TMJ and facial pain, pain in joints that are bone on bone, fibromyalgia pain, neuropathic pain, and pain after surgery or trauma.

1. I practice miracle medicine.

People often ask me, "What types of medicine do you practice?" I don't say it to be smart, but I say, "I practice miracle medicine." I'm referring to the miracles that happen with people who are told they have to have a hip replacement, but they're too old and that their heart's too weak. They cannot have surgery and are going to have to live with their condition. I work with them. We regrow the cartilage and strengthen the knee. They're walking

up and down the stairs again or living independently. They don't need to go to the nursing home. Those are the types of miracles that happen.

Everybody needs to know that just because an MRI reveals a torn meniscus does not mean that you have to have surgery. Arthroscopic surgery for that meniscus will not strengthen your knee and stop the osteoarthritis. A prolotherapy injection and Prolozone injections will do that. They'll stop osteoarthritis or degeneration of your joints cold when this process is completed.

When a new patient contacts my office for treatment of a complex musculoskeletal pain problem, my office will mail the person a new patient packet and schedule an office visit usually within two weeks. When I see the new patient, they will have filled out the history of their chief complaints including the treatments and medicines that they have tried. They will have given me a history of all their surgeries and completed a body chart, marking areas of injuries, fractures, surgical sites, or discomfort. The patient will also bring their bottles of medications and nutritional supplements and a completed review of all the systems of the body.

I then review all this information as well as any x-rays or laboratory reports. I question the patient to fill in the details of their history, and I personally review their dental history. This is often critical information that doctors neglect. A chronic bite problem or TMJ problem or a bone infection around a tooth can interfere with a patient's therapy.

I start my physical examination with the patient standing in their bare feet in front of me. I want to see the arches of their feet and how they're standing. I will examine and test their limbs, both the injured and healthy. I will examine the bones of the skull, including inside the mouth, and will treat "traumatic imprints" and blockages to movement as I go along.

We work our way up. It's interesting what patients have said to me. They have said, "My other doctor never examined my shoulder. He never had me take my shirt off. He sent me for X-rays and an MRI." They've never had someone put their hands on the body or do a range of motion tests. Another thing that may be a little different is so many doctors jump into the MRI and rely on the tests. There are many things I can tell are wrong with a joint just by my motion testing and getting the history. I'll say, "We have an unstable joint here. That's what needs to be fixed, not the diagnosis on the MRI." The other thing I say is that, "An MRI is not necessary in this case. An alternative is orthopedic ultrasound. The muscles and the tendons show up well, and it is much less expensive than an MRI." Many people have never heard that ultrasound could be used to examine a shoulder, a knee, or an ankle.

I then sit down with the patient and use models, anatomic pictures, x-rays, and lab work to show them what I've found to be the problem. I will also lay out my systematic treatment plan, explaining how each component works to help their body heal. Before I start any type of treatment, I may ask the patient to agree to stop certain medications and herbs, typically baby aspirin and Flexeril, a common muscle relaxant. These medications poison platelets, which they need in order to heal themselves.

It's very typical for the older population to be on a statin drug, which I strongly believe is an immune suppressant and promotes aches and pains in the body, as well as aspirin therapy, which we know causes you to urinate out more of your zinc. Statin drugs can be a source of pain, and they can also negatively affect the cell membranes of every muscle in the body, even muscles in the eye. I have had two patients whose vision improved once they had stopped their statin. The drug Singulair and the commonly used herbs curcumin and boswellia must be stopped because they block specific spots in the healing cascade of the body.

If the patient must stop medication and herbs first, I will not be able to perform Prolotherapy or inject Platelet Rich Plasma (PRP) for the regrowth of ligaments, tendons, and cartilage for three weeks. But I can start improving the range of motion and self-healing ability of the body with Mesotherapy. This is the injection of homeopathic medicine into the layer just under the skin (the mesoderm). Usually I will see instant improvement in the body's range of motion and a decrease in pain.

I will then follow this up with carefully applied neurotherapy, the injection of dilute lidocaine into all scars and any interference fields I have identified, and oftentimes around the skull. I frequently see instant pain relief, followed by fading of discolored scars, decreased edema of limbs, and improved function of limbs.

When Prolotherapy (the injection of sclerosing solution to stimulate the natural healing cascades of the body) is administered into and around a joint, a written guideline is given to the patient to instruct them on what supplements to take to help this process. When extra cartilage is desired in a joint I will add an injection of certain homeopathic medicine and ozone gas to stimulate growth. I have been doing this successfully since 1987. So you see, osteopathy takes a very broad perspective of the patient and applies all sciences to its understanding of the patient and is guided by its principles in the treatments that are used.

I'll do that similar type of orthopedic exam, which I call an osteopathic exam if someone is coming in and they have a hormone problem or a thyroid problem. I want to check the structure over, too. That's one thing that they'll perhaps find different. They've never had anyone be that thorough in examining them.

That gives you an idea of how I conduct an initial exam. You'd get a nutritional consultation, and we'd go over the medicines. I have a lot of models and pictures there. I sit next to the patient or have the husband and wife pull their chairs up next to each other. I use a skeleton with some pictures and say, "This is what a tendon is. This is what a ligament is. This is what a disc is. This is what your back looks like. This is where the problem is. This is how I fix it. Here's about how many treatments I think it will take. This is where we need to start."

I've had a number of patients say, "No one has ever told me what my problem's been. No one ever has explained it to me. I was told there's nothing more that can be done for me. I just have to learn to live with disability, this pain, and these pain pills or pain patches." I like it when I get those cases. Sometimes they'll say, after the first visit, "Oh my gosh, I started feeling better. You also gave me some hope."

DR. KONDROT: I like your approach. It's really interesting that you first look at the structure. Most doctors don't do that. They just go right to the X-ray or lab test. When you do examine somebody's structure starting with the feet and working your way up, what things do you look for that may give you some indication about their overall health or that can point to a particular disease?

DR. NEBBELING: One thing I look for in the feet is an arch or pronated feet. Do they stand with both toes pointing forward or are they rotated outward? With pronated feet, due to the force of gravity going up the leg, that person has abnormal force on their knees, lower back and even on their neck. I've sometimes had arch supports made for patients. It improved their headaches. It wasn't the total answer, but part of the stress on their body trying to balance themselves against gravity promoted headaches and muscular tension.

If we see shiny skin or loss of hair on the outside of the calves, the person may have reduced testosterone. We look at his age and any medication. With low hormones the patient will not respond as well to my other therapies.

When a person comes in and their feet or hands are cold and I see dry skin on their elbows, I'm thinking that this person has low metabolism. They may have a thyroid problem. They may not be blatantly hypothyroid, but they may have what we call subclinical hypothyroid. They would benefit from some iodine and some herbs, or maybe they need a small amount of natural thyroid or bioidentical thyroid to boost their metabolism. Every cell in the body is a receptor for thyroid hormone.

Many people seek me out just for that. They say, "Doctor, I've read these books and articles. It looks like I'm hypothyroid, but my doctor says that my tests are just fine and I don't have a problem." The physical exam, however, may point to a problem. This could lead me to want to look deeper and maybe do some lab testing and some other things.

DR. KONDROT: What are some of your favorite treatments that really make a

difference and that you feel more people should become aware of.

2. People do not have to live with pain and arthritis as long as their body possesses enough healing ability to heal itself.

DR. NEBBELING: Prolotherapy and Prolozone are injection techniques that stimulate the body to regrow ligaments tendons and cartilage. Prolotherapy is a proven medical technique that can result in stronger pain-free joints. I have successfully applied it to thousands of patients since 1987.

Second is Mesotherapy. Mesotherapy is a holistic injection technique that I feel the public should be aware of. This therapy was discovered and developed by a French physician in the 1950s. It involves the injection of small amounts of medicine just under the skin into the mesoderm. Mesotherapy was developed as a holistic therapy meaning it is not merely intended for cosmetic or pain purposes. It can be used to treat and balance all systems of the body thereby offering an alternative to the use of expensive, possibly dangerous, pharmaceuticals. I personally only use homeopathic preparations. I use Mesotherapy for pain and musculoskeletal problems, but I also address liver, digestive, adrenal, and depression problems.

Lastly, I would like to share what I can do for the aging population of people who have survived polio. I have a large group of very thankful post-polio patients. For those people who hyperextend and lock out their knee to walk, I utilize Prolozone to regrow cartilage in the knee and Prolotherapy to strengthen the ligaments. For patients who have worn out their wrists, elbows, and shoulders using crutches or pushing themselves up and out of a wheelchair, I rebuild those joints with Prolotherapy to keep them living independently. In those patients who previously have had tendon surgeries to their feet and ankle, I do neurotherapy to the painful scars and Prolozone to regrow cartilage in the ankle. All post-polio patients fear the flu or upper respiratory tract infections. Some remember being in the "Iron Lung" as a child and may have had a friend in their support group put on a respirator before they died. I use several methods of Oxidative Medicine to treat this concern. In doing so, I offer an alternative to vaccinations and common antibiotics for urinary tract and upper respiratory infections that frequently cause significant muscle weakness, making it necessary for the patients to recover in a nursing home.

I offer nebulized hydrogen peroxide solutions for patients to use in home for treatment and prevention of flu, colds, and lung infections. I treat respiratory infections in my office with intravenous hydrogen peroxide, photoluminescence, and ozone gas. I treat muscle weakness with Hyperbaric Oxygen Therapy (HBOT) in which a patient lies in a pressurized chamber with oxygen.

We inject certain medicines, which we make up in our office to cause controlled inflammation by the joints. That stimulates regrowth of ligaments, tendons, and cartilage. I also add Prolozone or inject some ozone and homeopathics into the joint to stimulate the cartilage and ligaments to grow.

I might integrate something known as neurotherapy or use a special type of compounded anesthetic and inject it where scar tissue is or where there are interference fields for healing in the body.

There's a whole area called oxidative therapies. I use those because they enhance my results with complex musculoskeletal cases. I've had people who had several joints that were bad or had several surgeries or had been in multiple car wrecks. Those people's responses are enhanced with oxidative therapies.

3. I've developed a special protocol for those with emphysema or COPD.

One of those areas that falls into oxidative therapy would be hydrogen peroxide. It's been used in medicine since World War I. British troops used it intravenously to help people who were infected by the flu. It was very successful for that. One thing I'd like the public to know is that it's very beneficial for anybody with emphysema or COPD. There's a special protocol I've developed where these patients come on a daily basis for two weeks. They have tremendous benefits to their condition, even people who have been on oxygen daily and are unable to leave their oxygen container. We've had people be able to stay off of it for several hours at a time and travel or do some activities of daily living without dependence on their oxygen.

Another part of oxidative therapy is the use of ozone gas. Medical ozone has wonderful benefits. It promotes the release of oxygen in our body. It up-regulates enzymes for us to make more energy. We see wonderful things happen with that. Of course, I do use ozone in my Prolozone. Some of that can be injected in a knee that no longer has any cartilage. When you're told you're bone-on-bone, it has wonderful results for that.

It also can be injected into the body in another way. That is another modality called photoluminescence or ultraviolet blood irradiation. We're actually able to treat any viruses or infections in the blood. It's very good for people who have chronic fatigue syndrome or multiple mixed bacterial infections, and even people with unhealed bone infections. That is an oxidative therapy for the blood.

It has wonderful benefits in balancing our nervous system and stimulating the immune system, as well as deactivating toxins and helping us fight bacterial infections and viruses in our body. It has wonderful applications for many things, from hepatitis C infections, to MRSA infections, and unhealed bone infections, but also for chronic fatigue syndrome, people with asthma, and some autoimmune diseases such as rheumatoid arthritis.

DR. KONDROT: Could you comment on how you select the oxidative treatment, typically how many therapies a patient will need, and when they will notice an improvement. Is this something where you do one treatment, or do you have to do a series of 20 or 30 treatments?

DR. NEBBELING: That's an excellent question. For those of us who are trained in oxidative medicine, the modalities we tend to have are hydrogen peroxide and hyperbaric oxygen. I will start with my NebuMist program, which is a specially formulated liquid containing hydrogen peroxide (H_2O_2). A small amount of this solution is placed in the medicine cup of a nebulizer (asthma machine). The nebulizer converts the solution into microscopic bubbles that can be inhaled deeply into the lungs, thoroughly treating diseases like emphysema and infections like influenza, viral pneumonia, bacterial pneumonia, and more. I believe every home in America should have a nebulizer and bag of H_2O_2 in their refrigerator. It can be used once a day as prevention or every half hour for treatment of an acute cold or sinus infection. For a cold, symptomatic improvement is often seen after a day of treatment. Intravenous H_2O_2 has many benefits for my patients. It boosts immune function, kills invading organisms such as viruses, bacteria, fungus, and parasites. It also dilates the arteries and veins.

If I could think of one kind of patient who responds well to H_2O_2, it would be those with emphysema or COPD. I have treated patients in the early stages, who are just short of breath and use an inhaler, and I have treated end-stage patients who are hospitalized once or more per year and have not been off their oxygen in over two years. I have the patient commit to daily treatments for two weeks. After the ten intravenous treatments I send them home with the NebuMist program. Every patient notices improvement within the first week, many after the first treatment!

Hyperbaric Oxygen Therapy (HBOT) is a technology that delivers oxygen to the body while under pressure. The patient lies down in the chamber (it feels like being in a pup tent), the door is zipped shut and sealed. Then a compressor pressurizes the chamber. The treatment lasts one hour. The patients who especially benefit from HBOT are those with multiple sclerosis (MS). I believe that when first diagnosed with MS, one should get 20 treatments of HBOT. The next group of patients would be anyone who is having mini strokes called TIA or anyone who has had a stroke. I've had patients who have had strokes who within one or two treatments would say, "I'm able to button my blouse now without looking down at it." They are able to drive and do other things. Their fine motor skills had returned in one or two treatments. One woman had not spoken for four years after her stroke. After her first hyperbaric treatment, she started speaking again. Results can happen very fast. That's the miracle of medicine. Some of my

patients have seen benefits after just one treatment. However, many patients need more than ten.

Photoluminescence therapy in my office is the removal of a quantity of blood from the body, washing the blood with ozone gas and then subjecting it to ultraviolet light. The process was originally called Ultraviolet Blood Irradiation (UBI). There are enough documented benefits from UBI that I would recommend everybody receive four treatments a year as prevention. However, a few patients who have amazing benefits from UBI are those with non-healing antibiotic-resistant bone infections. It is also beneficial for those suffering from chronic fatigue syndrome. Then I would mention a very important group of patients: adults with Chronic Lymphocytic Leukemia (CLL). Toward the end of the disease, the patient's body will start to make a large number of cancer cells. At that point, they must undergo chemotherapy or die. It has been our experience that if late stage CLL patients receive UBI treatments they can avoid "Blast Crisis" and chemotherapy for years.

DR. KONDROT: These are really amazing stories. The question I have is after you do a series of ten or more oxidative treatments, how long do these treatments last? Does the patient have to come back to have a repeat session, or is it permanent?

DR. NEBBELING: That's a good question. For an MS patient who has had 20

HBOT, the research seems to show that that's a permanent benefit. For COPD patients who have received ten intravenous H2O2 treatments, many of them are maintained satisfactorily at home on the NebuMist program, although they may come back occasionally for one or two intravenous treatments, if they wish. For patients with bone infections, once they have finished their UBI treatments, it is a permanent cure. I have followed up with patients five and six years later, and the infection has not returned. For a stroke patient who recovers function after a series of HBOT treatments, this is a permanent benefit. They then move on to other preventative treatments.

A person with COPD may maintain and be satisfied with the therapy. They have permanent lung damage, usually due to smoking cigarettes. These people will benefit if they maintain themselves with the home therapy of breathing the hydrogen peroxide in. That can be a permanent benefit.

Perhaps someone has seasonal allergies, and they get the photoluminescence treatment. They would get four treatments in a row separated by one day. They'll often go for a year. They may come back in a year and say, "I'd like another tune-up, Dr. Nebbeling." They receive benefits for their allergy symptoms for up to a year after a series of four treatments.

DR. KONDROT: That's truly remarkable. Now, please discuss how you are helping people with chronic eye problems. You were recently trained at the Florida Eye and Wellness Center on some of the latest techniques I'm using to help people with macular degeneration, glaucoma, and other eye problems.

DR. NEBBELING: It was interesting that we were already doing all the modalities needed to treat the eye, except the microcurrent machine, which you introduced to me, but we were applying them for different needs. We weren't applying them to help improve the eye. It wasn't a very big jump to this, however, as you explained things to me. I just applied the osteopathic philosophy to the person's health. If there is uninterrupted nerve flow and good blood supply, you find health and healing.

The retina is one big area of blood vessels, and the optic nerve is the second cranial nerve coming out of the brain. It's a big nerve. If we can detoxify it, get more oxygen, improve blood supply, and get more nutrition to it, we'll be able to see changes.

The things I didn't know were how to diagnose problems with the eye and how to measure the outcomes and improvements. You've helped train me this past year to get good records beforehand and to do proper testing before we start things.

We do heavy metal testing and provocative heavy metal challenges when everybody comes here. Then we start detoxifying the patient and giving them the microcurrent treatments. We also do the light therapy you've taught me how to apply to patients. For the past two years, every patient who has come through here has had some improvement within three days, all the way up to amazing improvement. One young man with retinitis pigmentosa said, "I feel like I'm seeing behind my head now," because he didn't realize how narrow his field of vision was.

DR. KONDROT: You're essentially using many of these modalities for other chronic disease. It's just a natural progression for you to now use them for a different part of the body. All the body parts are connected. By strengthening the foundation, you essentially strengthen all the organ systems. It's truly miracle medicine. Maybe you could go into a little bit more detail about your eye therapy program.

DR. NEBBELING: It usually starts off with a phone call to us. We get the basic demographic material on the patient and request recent eye records. If the patient does not have them, we get those ordered. We really need to know what the person has. Once we receive those records, we forward them to Dr. Kondrot, who will develop the program and then send those parts of the program to me to administer.

In the meantime, if the patient is close enough, we schedule a new patient office visit. It starts off similarly to what I described for my other patients. They will bring in all their vitamins, minerals, and medicines, and I'll do a physical examination. If there's time, we will have ordered

lab work because I want to know what the kidney function is. If we're going to do heavy metal testing, we'll need to know that.

We test for toxins through urine tests, first in a pretest to see the background exposure to toxins. Then we give two chelators intravenously, followed by some glutathione, a potent antioxidant. Then the patient collects their urine for six hours. The lab analyzes it for the presence of about a dozen toxic minerals. That's the best, latest way of testing things.

The three-day program includes ozonated eye drops and a liquid mineral supplement. We start building up the nutritional status and adding some oxygen and oxidative properties to the eyes. We also do vascular testing to see how the blood flow is in the extremities. As we see improvements in the blood flow to the rest of the body, we infer how that affects the eye. We'll do a zinc taste test, and then we actually give some intravenous minerals.

Eye patients get the IV photoluminescence as well as hyperbaric oxygen chamber treatments. They get hydrogen peroxide on one of the three days. We consider the ozonated eye drops another oxidative therapy. All in all, we work with eyes and vision the same way we work with other problems in the body, holistically and according to osteopathic principles.

....

DAVID P NEBBELING, DO
Advanced Osteopathic Health
3918 W. St. Joseph Hwy
Lansing, MI 48917
517-323-1833
www.davidnebbelingdo.com

Karl Robinson, MD

HOUSTON, TEXAS

August 25, 2013

1. Homeopathy – The incredible power of small doses

2. Homeopathy – The subtle medicine that produces seismic change

3. Homeopathy – The only medical system that treats the mental, emotional, and physical at one time with one medicine

DR. KONDROT: Today my guest is an exceptional alternative doctor whom I greatly respect. His specialty is homeopathy. He is Dr. Karl Robinson whom I consider to be one of my homeopathic teachers. I wanted to begin by having you share a little bit about your medical career and how you became interested in homeopathy.

DR. ROBINSON: I'm a graduate of Hahnemann Medical College of Philadelphia, the same medical school that you also went to. Then I did a residency in New York City at Harlem Hospital where I became rather disillusioned with conventional medicine and started looking around.

In the course of the next year or so, I started learning about homeopathy and then took my first course. After that I started studying all over the world, learning from top-rate homeopaths in virtually every country where homeopathy is practiced: England, Belgium, Holland, the United States, Canada, India, and Argentina. I continue to this day studying because homeopathy is not so easy to master, and it is eternally fascinating. Currently, I try to go to Mumbai,

India, once or twice a year to study with Prafull Vijayakar, a great prescriber.

DR. KONDROT: That's one thing I really admire about you. Homeopathy is a very difficult discipline, and it seems like you're never satisfied. You're always pursuing a different teacher and a different approach. I think as a result of all of this, you have sharpened your skills and improved your technique in case taking and analysis over the years.

Before we talk about that, one of the biggest problems is actually explaining homeopathy. There are so many misconceptions. I'm going to ask if you could explain to us what exactly homeopathy is. I'm sorry to put you on the spot. It can be very difficult to do this in a short time.

1. The incredible power of small doses

DR. ROBINSON: Homeopathy is the brainchild of Dr. Samuel Hahnemann, a German who lived over 200 years ago. It's based on a principle he discovered which is that anything a substance can cause in the way of symptoms, that same substance in a small dose can take those symptoms away. A small example: If, when cutting up onions, your eyes, and nose water as they also do in colds and allergic conditions, then a tiny dose of that same onion can take away those symptoms. In fact, a homeopathic preparation of the onion known as *Allium cepa* can be used to treat those very symptoms.

The only therapy outside of homeopathy which is slightly similar is allergy treatments where people get injections of the allergen that they're allergic to in order to desensitize them. That's quite a crude form of what homeopathy does.

When we treat people, we use a single medicine and that medicine invariably affects the mind, the intellect, and the emotions. It almost always affects all organs and systems of the body, so in one medicine we have the ability to affect the mind, the emotions, and the body. You can see, then, that homeopathic medicine has a much broader scope than allergy desensitization.

When we are with a sick person, we are listening for symptoms, which correspond to one of the medicines that we've already investigated. When we find a match between the patient's symptoms and one of the homeopathic medicines whose various therapeutic qualities are known, then we give that medicine. We homeopaths call this the Law of Similars which means we use the homeopathic medicine most similar to the symptoms the patient presents with. Of course, we give it in a micro dosage. When we have a really good match between the homeopathic medicine and the patient's various symptoms, the patient will begin to improve in a global sort of way. That is to say, different problems will resolve.

2. The subtle medicine that produces seismic changes

Say the person has high blood pressure, irritable bowel, and headaches. The right homeopathic medicine will clear up all three problems. I know it sounds a bit fantastic as conventional medicine routinely treats the hypertension with an antihypertensive, the headaches with one or more analgesics, and the irritable bowel with an antispasmodic. Yet, routinely, we find that one homeopathic medicine, carefully selected, will work on all aspects of the person. We can therefore say, homeopathy is truly *holistic* as mind and body are being put into order by *one* medicine *at the same time.*

If a person has a recurrent sinus problem and we learn that they also have or have had stomach ulcers, there's only one homeopathic medicine which covers both sinus infections and stomach ulcers, and that's *Kali bichromicum,* the bichromate of potassium.

In this way, we're able to join together quite separate organs and systems which are dysfunctional with one homeopathic medicine, and, when that homeopathic medicine is carefully prescribed, we see not just one problem get better but several. One looks for a general improvement in the energy, mind, and disposition as well as an improvement in the physical problems. Many times we'll find more than one physical problem gets better, which is quite astounding. Does that give you an idea?

DR. KONDROT: It's interesting because it's so different from traditional Western medicine. If you have a sinus problem, you go to an ear, nose, and throat doctor, and he will treat the sinuses. If you have

stomach ulcers, you go to a gastroenterologist, and he will treat that separate part of the body.

What you're saying in homeopathy is that you're treating the whole person. Could you explain how homeopathy works when you're treating different parts of the body? It's contrary to traditional Western medicine.

DR. ROBINSON: The unifying concept, which comes straight from Samuel Hahnemann, is that when people fall ill, there is this subtle energy which surrounds and penetrates the body which gets discombobulated or out of joint. Hahnemann called this the Vital Force. Some people might prefer to call it, chi, (ch'i) or something else, but Hahnemann called it the Vital Force, so we'll stay with that.

The idea is that the Vital Force, in disease, is out of order and it's not flowing in a uniform and healthy way. These homeopathic medicines are very subtle in themselves. They've been highly diluted and "succussed" which means shaken vigorously. When we find the correct homeopathic medicine, we believe that it unblocks this disordered energy field, the Vital Force. When the homeopathic medicine puts the Vital Force into a balanced or normal state, the now healthy Vital Force exerts a beneficial influence on the body, physically, chemically, and physiologically, allowing it to cure itself. In a way, you could say that homeopathy promotes self-healing. Think of a magnet and how it will cause iron filings to line up; that is a crude analogy to how the Vital Force acts.

DR. KONDROT: I wonder if you could talk a little bit about *Belladonna* and use that as an example to illustrate some of the points that you covered so far about different organ systems improving.

DR. ROBINSON: *Belladonna* is used in conventional medicine as an antispasmodic and that's about it. It calms down spasms that occur in the gut.

Used homeopathically it has a wide range of actions, and in the homeopathic investigations, which we call *provings*, it was found that *Belladonna*, when given to healthy persons, acts on the circulatory system in a very specific way. It promotes an uneven distribution of the blood, forcing it upward into the head and neck and away from the extremities. In these provings of *Belladonna,* we find that the hands and feet are noticeably cooler than the face and head. At the same time, *Belladonna* causes the pupils of the eye to dilate or enlarge.

Because of the increased circulation upward, you'll notice that the large arteries in the neck, known as the carotid arteries, are visibly pulsating. If you hold your hand about eight to ten inches above the person's face, you'll feel heat radiating upward.

This corresponds to a number of fevers that children get. They'll spike a fever which will rise rather quickly up to 103 degrees, 104 degrees, or even 105 degrees. With the fever, you'll find that the face will go red as well as become hot. If you run your hands down to the hands and feet, you'll find that they're noticeably cooler.

The interesting thing is when you find this particular conjunction of symptoms, *Belladonna* will be indicated in *several different* clinical presentations. For example, it will be useful in a simple fever, pharyngitis (sore throat), tonsillitis, and otitis media, which is infection of the middle ear. It has even proved useful in meningitis, although I don't suggest you just treat it only with homeopathy. You should also get the kid to the hospital.

When this particular group of symptoms is present, all these different clinical presentations usually resolve in short order with homeopathic treatment. It's quite extraordinary when you consider that with conventional medicine, if you have otitis, you're going to be given an antibiotic and an analgesic, whereas *Belladonna* will take care of both the pain and the inflammation in the middle ear. Not only that, but it will bring the fever down often within minutes or an hour or so. You have one medicine, then, capable of treating three, four, or five different clinical presentations. That's pretty amazing. There's nothing conventional medicine can point to that can do the same thing. Remember, however, that the symptoms must match *Belladonna*. We have hundreds of other medicines each with a different set of actions. The idea, always, is to select the homeopathic medicine most similar to the presenting symptoms of the patient.

DR. KONDROT: I wonder if you could talk more about how a homeopathic remedy treats different organs and systems. You talked about *Belladonna* treating the ear problem. When that same presentation occurs in a different part of the body, such as in a sore throat or abscess, *Belladonna* might be useful. I wonder if you could clarify how this could happen.

DR. ROBINSON: Let's say a nursing mother develops mastitis which is an infection of the breast. If it's a *Belladonna* case, you would note that the affected part of the breast feels hot to the patient, and it is hot to the touch. Touching the area would also be quite painful, and it would be throbbing or pulsating.

Remember, I said that *Belladonna* causes the carotid artery to pulsate. It can cause pulsation anywhere there is inflammation such as a cellulitis or an abscess. There is also redness, often swelling, and tenderness. Anywhere in the body that you have inflammation with these signs, you could be looking at case in which *Belladonna* could prove curative.

DR. KONDROT: Let's talk about another homeopathic medicine that maybe has a different presentation from *Belladonna* to illustrate the powers of homeopathy and how homeopathy can affect many different organ systems and parts of the body.

DR. ROBINSON: I'll say a few words about *Opium*, which is made by diluting and succussing the opiate. Now, before you freak, remember that opium, the opiate, has been diluted beyond the point where any molecules remain. It is entirely energetic, not chemical. Homeopathic *Opium*, like the narcotic it once was, is useful for people who can tolerate quite a bit more pain than usual. Other symptoms of *Opium* are sleepiness to the point where they look and act dopey and an indifference to their surroundings. Some people needing homeopathic *Opium* act like zombies. Their pupils are usually dilated. Perhaps most interesting is the fact this state usually comes on as the result of a great fright or shock. Say the person was in a motor vehicle accident and immediately or soon after went into the state described above. *Opium* would restore him or her to the pre-shock state. Clearly, *Opium* is one of our primo medicines for post-traumatic stress disorder (PTSD). This is true even if the traumatic event occurred weeks, months, or years earlier.

I have treated numerous patients with *Opium* over the years, often with astonishing results. One was a 19-year-old woman who had been in a daze virtually all her life. It dated from her birth, which had been frightening and utterly traumatic to her mother. (See my website: www. homeopathyyes.com "Lifelong depression in a 19-year-old woman — cured with *Opium*.") Somehow, the fright and trauma of the birth got imprinted onto the baby affecting her entire nervous system and lasting for 19 years.

After a single dose of *Opium*, she came out of her 19-yearlong trance as though awakening from an endless Rip Van Winkle type sleep. Within three weeks, she found a job, and then went on to marry and have a child. Best of all, she became energetic and happy.

I should mention that there are numerous medicines for persons suffering from physical and/or emotional trauma, not only *Opium*. Some of the more useful are *Stramonium, Arnica, Aconite,* and *Gelsemium*. Each has a different constellation of symptoms even though all treat PTSD. It is my strong conviction that homeopathic medicine could help immensely the thousands of soldiers who served in Iraq and Afghanistan and who now suffer from PTSD.

Let's also mention *Rhus toxicodendron*, which is poison ivy. When it's prepared homeopathically, it becomes an important medicine for ligaments, joints, and muscles.

The symptomatology of *Rhus toxicodendron* is quite interesting because people with muscle and joint problems will tell you invariably that on waking in the morning or after they've been seated for a long time, when they first move, they feel a lot of stiffness and pain. That's one of the cardinal symptoms of *Rhus toxicodendron*. They're worse after being at rest for a while.

When they say, "It's very hard for me to take a trip of 100 or 200 miles, so I have to stop every 30 or 40 minutes to get out and stretch," that's because the joints, ligaments, and muscles feel worse when they're not moving.

Ironically, the first movements hurt, but after they warm up, a lot of people with arthritis will say, "It's really bad for the first few steps, but after I walk for a while or take a hot shower, I start to feel better."

Rhus toxicodendron is better from heat. It is also sensitive to the approach of a storm, so you'll hear people say, "I can sense when a thunderstorm or change of weather is coming even when it's 100 or 200 miles away. I begin to feel it. I begin to ache." That's another sign of *Rhus toxicodendron*.

Rhus toxicodendron is better not after the first movement but continued movement, but it's more complicated than that. If they keep moving, at the end of the day they'll start to feel pain again. It's worse from the first movement and better from continued movement, up to a point. Then they feel worse again. Again, I should caution, *Rhus toxicodendron* does not work for all joint or ligament pains. We have many, many homeopathic medicines which may be indicated depending on the *totality of the symptoms*, a phrase that Hahnemann coined, meaning the most important mental, emotional, *and* physical symptoms taken together.

DR. KONDROT: When a patient sees you for a physical problem, is their emotional state important? How do you sort that out?

DR. ROBINSON: That is a most interesting question.

3. The only medical system that treats the mental, emotional and physical at one time with one medicine

A classic situation is a middle-aged woman who complains of migraines. My first question is always, "When did they start?" Often, she'll mention a specific time some years back. I'll then ask, "What was going on in your life just before the migraines started?" At that point, she might very well say that her son was killed in Iraq and begin to weep.

Now, I'm at the meat of the matter. Her migraines are a manifestation of unresolved grief. I say, "unresolved," because she still weeps, years later, and I have just learned that the migraines came on shortly after her son's death. So, I know I'll need a medicine for grief *and* headaches. I further learn, by careful questioning, that when she is sad or unhappy, she dislikes people fussing over her. "I hate that," she'll say. "I'd rather deal with my grief alone." Also, if she goes out into the hot sun, it will trigger a migraine within 15 to 20 minutes. Finally, I learn that she craves salt and salty foods.

This particular complex of symptoms:

1. Unresolved grief,

2. Worse from consolation,

3. Headaches from exposure to the sun, and

4. Desire for salt

point to one medicine only and that is *Natrum muriaticum*, which is Latin for sodium chloride or salt. I give it in a homeopathic dose, and, when I see her a month later, both her grief *and* her migraines will be considerably better and will entirely go away in a few months. So, in answer to your question, the classical homeopath always looks for clues in the emotional sphere as well as the physical. Such a constellation of symptoms is, as I mentioned earlier, the *totality of symptoms.*

Gathering this totality takes time and, in the initial visit, I spend up to an hour and a half with an adult or an hour with a child. This history involves not only the complaint or complaints, because there are often more than one, but also includes things like how the person reacts to all kinds of environmental stimuli.

Let me give you some examples. We want to know: Is the person hot or cold? Does she tolerate cold or not? Is she thirsty or thirstless? If thirsty, does she want cold, room temperature, or hot drinks? Is she affected by weather? Are there any foods that she craves or dislikes or that make her ill? We want to know if the patient perspires and if there's anything unusual about the perspiration. We go into great detail.

Then we get to the emotional side. Very often, people fall ill after either a single great stress or a series of stresses. A chronically ill woman with multiple problems might tell how, when she was little, she lived in fear of her father who was alcoholic. He would come home drunk late at night, wake her, and sometimes abuse her. Much of her childhood was spent in a state of intense fear. When I see her years later, she is chronically ill with a spate of both physical and emotional problems. In order to make her better, the homeopathic medicine must address her terror as well as her physical problems.

DR. KONDROT: I have a couple of questions for you. First, how does someone find a well-trained, competent homeopathic doctor? Also, what are the sources of homeopathic education in the United States?

DR. ROBINSON: To learn about homeopathy, one of the first steps is to go online to the National Center for Homeopathy (NCH). They have a website, nationalcenterforhomeopathy.org and maintain a database of homeopaths around the country. If you join the NCH, they have a magazine which is quite interesting that comes out every couple of months, and they have an annual conference.

Perhaps the best place to find a good doctor is through the American Institute of Homeopathy (AIH) homeopathyusa.org which is an organization for MDs and DOs who practice homeopathy.

These two organizations will enable you to learn more about homeopathy as well as to find a homeopath. There are also schools throughout the United States that offer training in homeopathy. Several naturopathic colleges include homeopathic education. There are some homeopathic schools that meet usually once a month for three or four days for one, two, or three years. That's another way to learn. Usually non-doctors attend these courses. All these can be found online.

There are many bookstores you can find online to buy books about homeopathy. Homeopathic Education Services, Nature-Reveals, and Bjain Books (India) are all excellent.

DR. KONDROT: I know that you're very modest, but you've been working on a book. It's an introductory book where you explain in detail the art and science of homeopathy. I wonder if you could tell us a little about it.

DR. ROBINSON: I'm interested in trying to educate the average person about the possibilities of homeopathic medicine. The book aims at those who are dissatisfied with conventional medicine and millions fall into the dissatisfied category. These folks need to know that homeopathy, in the hands of a skillful practitioner, can make a huge difference in all sorts of diseases including autoimmune, neurological, and metabolic diseases and many others. Many difficult issues that are not readily classified by conventional medicine can be helped and sometimes cured completely by homeopathy. To do this, you need somebody who really knows what he's doing.

Conventional medicine really cannot cure, that is, completely resolve, any chronic illness. At best, it can control and palliate chronic disease, but it cannot cure. I define a cure when the patient has no more complaints and needs *no medicine* whether pharmaceutical or homeopathic. In addition, he is full of energy and interested in his life.

DR. KONDROT: We tend to live in a very impatient society where we're used to quick fixes. One thing people have to understand with homeopathy is that often it's a slow process to regain health. I wonder if you could express some of your opinions on this aspect of homeopathy?

DR. ROBINSON: If it's an acute problem, we have to get them well pretty quickly.

The other day I treated a woman who had severe vertigo. I gave her one medicine that didn't work. The next day, 12 hours later, I prescribed a different medicine, and that one did work. Her vertigo calmed down significantly and quite rapidly. We can't just wait. You need to get a result, and you need to get it pretty quickly. That's with an acute problem.

If it's a chronic problem, it rarely goes away quickly. It may take weeks or months, and that's with the correct medicine. People have to understand that.

Often people come in to see a homeopath and they're on one, three, five, seven, or more different pharmaceutical medicines. We have to take a case history allowing for the fact that they're on all these drugs. This can be quite daunting because the various drugs, being so powerful, do not allow a clear glimpse of the underlying problems. The natural illness, then, is covered over. But we do our best. Then we prescribe and, hopefully, they start to feel better than they did on their drugs. As they improve, we begin slowly to take them off their drugs. We don't want to just take them off immediately because we don't want to put them in any danger. People have to realize that if you're suffering from a chronic problem, you're not going to get better overnight.

DR. KONDROT: When you go to a health food store, you can't help but see a lot of homeopathic products. The question I have is whether these homeopathic products can be helpful for common problems if a person does not have any training in the use of homeopathic medicines? Are they safer to use than traditional medication? Let's say you have a cold or flu, and you really don't want to take antibiotics, aspirin, or Tylenol. You want to explore homeopathy. I wonder if you could comment on how someone who may be hearing about homeopathy for the first time can get involved and begin to appreciate the value of homeopathy.

DR. ROBINSON: That's an interesting question. Fortunately or unfortunately, these homeopathic medicines have become widely available in health food stores. Whole Foods Market stocks them, as do many health food stores. They're available. Yes, they are safe. The problem with having them available is that it makes for a trivialization of homeopathy. People think, "I can pick up a homeopathic medicine for $3, $4, or $5." For them, homeopathy is on the same level as buying an herbal preparation or vitamins and minerals. They think, "I can treat myself." You have to be very skilled or very lucky when you buy your homeopathic medicine. If it works, mostly it's a matter of luck because it's not so simple.

For reasons which are unclear to me, the FDA requires homeopathic manufacturers to label each homeopathic medicine with one or two words. This is really bizarre because a homeopathic medicine like *Natrum muriaticum*, mentioned earlier, has over 2,000 symptoms in its proving. To reduce all that information to one or two words is ludicrous. But that's what the FDA insists on.

Some people use *Oscillococcinum*, a homeopathic medicine for the flu. It is made by Boiron, a French company, and it often works to reduce flu symptoms. Also, you can use *Arnica* for bruises and it will work, but when it comes to more complicated things, it's kind of a raffle. As I said, you have to be either very lucky or very knowledgeable to help in chronic illnesses.

DR. KONDROT: Dr. Robinson, I'm going to throw a pretty tough question at you. What, really, brings a patient to consult a homeopath, and how has conventional medicine failed him, and how is homeopathy different?

DR. ROBINSON: The first thing that has to happen is the person has to become disenchanted with modern medicine. That's what happened to me when I was a resident in Harlem Hospital in New York City. It started to dawn on me that the medicine I was being taught could do little other than palliate or alleviate the symptoms. Modern medicine, with its powerful chemical agents, forces the body to do what the doctor decrees. Antihypertensives force the blood pressure down; antiglycemics make the blood glucose fall; antianxiety agents knock the edge off the angst, and so on. In every case, the body is being forced to do what it has no inclination to do on its own.

Let me give you a typical example. Many people come in with multi-organ, multi-system illnesses. For example, they have migraines (brain/vascular) and hypertension (cardiovascular). Their sugar may be too high, and they're headed toward diabetes (endocrine). They have arthritic pains (musculoskeletal), a dermatitis (skin), constipation (gastrointestinal), and anxiety (mental/emotional). They have all these problems affecting all these organs and systems.

When they go the regular route, they get shunted here and there to various specialists, and they get placed on one or more medicines for the hypertension, one or more analgesics for the migraines, steroid ointment for the skin problem, an anti-inflammatory for the joints and something else for the constipation, and, of course, they'll receive an antianxiety pill. This approach divides the body into its components. Everything is segmented and, in the process, the person, her intricate and most interesting nature, gets left out. She, the person and her wonderfully complex life, is forgotten. Often she is reduced to the sum of her laboratory values, scans, and ultrasounds. Modern medicine has yet to learn that a sick person is a delicate web of thoughts and feelings, far more than the sum of her organ parts.

How different is homeopathy? With our broad, in-depth, and lengthy interview, we are curious about *all aspects* of the person. We note everything from her expressions to her gestures to the tone of her voice. We listen for recurring words and themes. We pay full attention to everything all the while working to find that one *most similar* homeopathic medicine which will address her and her multi-organ, multi-system illnesses.

I am not against modern medicine. Definitely, it has its place and I am glad it is there. There are situations in which it is life-saving and life-prolonging. It is when it fails to bring about health that we must look elsewhere and homeopathic medicine is a peerless alternative.

DR. KONDROT: I can speak personally about myself. I developed severe adult onset asthma. Traditional Western medicine was able to palliate or reduce my symptoms, but it did nothing in terms of curing the asthma. Of course, there were a lot of side effects to the drugs. It wasn't until I was introduced to homeopathy that my asthma was truly cured. That was 15 years ago, and I no longer need any type of asthma medication. That convinced me that the homeopathic approach is the best approach, but it's not simple or easy.

I'm sure you have the situation where people ask you, "What's the best homeopathic remedy for asthma or a headache?" They fail to understand we really don't treat disease, per se. We treat the whole person, so it takes quite a bit more work and effort. The end result is that you're going to be much healthier overall and less dependent on medications to maintain your system.

Dr. Robinson, I know one thing you're really interested in is improving the quality of homeopathic education and sharing the wonders of homeopathy with the traditional medical system. Do you think traditional medicine will ever embrace homeopathy?

DR. ROBINSON: Up to this point, it's a bit of a pipe dream. We hope it will, but I don't hold my breath. As I said a minute ago, they have this very specialized outlook that disease localizes, affecting various parts of the body. We have all these specialists. They don't seem to grasp that it's impossible for only one part of the body to fall ill. A human being is a seamless whole. It's as though we are one very complicated mobile. Set one part in motion, and the whole contraption begins to sway and move. It is all interconnected. When people fall ill, the mind, the emotions, *and* the body are all affected. Currently, regular medicine only pays lip service to this reality. It either cannot or does not want to acknowledge the profound interconnectedness that each person is.

For the conventionally trained doctor, it is incomprehensible that I could successfully treat a child with both seizures and asthma with one dose of one homeopathic medicine. Yet, I did and then watched as *both* the seizures and the asthma got better and disappeared. (See the case on my website: "Seizures and asthma both cured with one homeopathic medicine.")

One has to understand what's possible with homeopathy and what's not possible with conventional medicine.

DR. KONDROT: I wonder if you could share with us a little about your current practice, also, your involvement with homeopathic education in Central America.

DR. ROBINSON: I'm primarily stationed in Houston, Texas. I travel frequently to El Salvador and to Guatemala where I teach. In 2014, I'll be in my 12th year in those countries. Prior to that, I taught

in Honduras, and, before that, a bit in Cuba. I am doing my best to spread homeopathy. Together with another MD, I founded the Texas Society of Homeopathy. We hold a conference once a year.

DR. KONDROT: If people are interested in your book, *Small Doses, Big Results – How Homeopathic Medicine Offers Hope in Chronic Disease*, www.amazon.com will list it. They can also contact your website and office for more information.

We have a few minutes left in the show. I wonder if you could give the listeners some advice on bringing homeopathy into their lives.

DR. ROBINSON: I have devoted my entire professional life to the study and practice of homeopathy, and it's been entirely satisfying. Every patient is different. I don't care if you have a common diagnosis. You are in some way different from everyone else with the same diagnosis. We take that into account.

You are a person who is unique, and you need a unique medicine to treat you mentally, emotionally, and physically. We're not treating you in a routine way. We're trying to treat all aspects of you at one time. For us, your diagnosis is only the first step in finding the most similar homeopathic medicine. I honestly believe that homeopathy is the only truly holistic medicine because, with one medicine, we take into account the enormously complex person in front of us.

....

KARL ROBINSON, MD
Houston, Texas
(713)621-3184.
www.homeopathyyes.com

Robert Rowen, MD, MD(H)

SANTA ROSA, CALIFORNIA

Interviewed September 8, 2013

1. **You can detox from mercury with supplements at home.**

2. **Chelation Therapy for heavy metals: now do it at home.**

3. **Oxidation Therapies can cure even fatal diseases!**

DR. KONDROT: This evening, we have a special treat. My good friend, Dr. Robert Rowen, is my guest. I always joke that when we take our yearly hike together, I probably learn more from him talking about alternative treatments on the trails than I do from all the medical meetings that I go to that year.

Let's get right into it. I'm sure a lot of the listeners are interested in a little bit about your medical career and how you got interested in alternative treatments, which eventually led you to writing one of the leading alternative newsletters in the country, *Second Opinion*, and to becoming a sought-after speaker all over the United States.

DR. ROWEN: The truth is that at the end of my third year of medical school at the University of California, San Francisco, I almost quit. I was really depressed because I saw patient after patient getting a battery of testing procedures, sometimes very invasive tests, and it all amounted to nothing because they either couldn't be treated, or they were treated with petrochemical drugs.

I wasn't aware that that was what medicine was all about when I walked into it. I thought we were about healing. As one who was very much against the toxic pollution of the planet, I came to see that we were treating our patients exactly as we were treating the planet, pouring chemicals into them. After I got out of medical school, I kept an open mind, looking for any way not to give people chemical medicine.

DR. KONDROT: Why are you so much against chemical medicine? There are pharmaceutical companies saying this is the solution to our health problems and that the petrochemicals will take care of all our needs.

DR. ROWEN: I'm not sure they're exactly saying that. You've seen me lecture before. I've lectured in international circles. Sometimes I'll hold up a huge piece of currency, like $100, and say, "I'll give this to the first one of you who can name me any synthetic petrochemical pharmaceutical, with the exception of antibiotics, that cures any disease." Guess how many takers I've had. Not one. I don't think God makes mistakes, and God didn't make any of us with an inherent genetic biological deficiency of a chemical that's not found in nature.

I want to clarify something you said. It's not that I'm against petrochemical medicine. I'm not. I think that for every chemical that's out there, there could potentially be a reason to use it. I said "potentially," but I think that 90% of the time or more, it shouldn't be used. Does that make sense?

DR. KONDROT: It does, but I wonder if you'll educate us in terms of side effects, dependencies, or harm petrochemicals

are causing with the body.

DR. ROWEN: Virtually every drug in pharma's armamentarium is an anti. It's antibiotic, anti-pain, analgesic, anti-inflammatory, and antihypertensive. It's anti this and anti that. Give me a break. Where do they have things that actually do something?

If it's an anti, it's inhibiting something. For example, with blood pressure, there's angiotensin converting enzyme inhibitors. For psychiatry, there's SSRIs, selective serotonin reuptake inhibitors. They're inhibitors; they're inhibiting function. Instead of inhibiting function, we should bring the body back into balance by giving it what it needs to be in balance.

Hold your left and your right arms above your head. Your hands are equal. Now bring your right arm down to shoulder level. You're out of balance. What pharma is doing is giving you a chemical to bring your left arm down to shoulder level instead of bringing your right arm back up for optimum functioning. Does that make sense?

DR. KONDROT: Yes, and you and I agree that the human body is very complex. By blocking one enzymatic reaction or treating one aspect, there could be a myriad of reactions that might potentially be harmful.

DR. ROWEN: I wouldn't even say "might potentially." I would say it's likely.

I'm going to give you some examples. Look at the Vioxx scandal. It's an anti-inflammatory. It inhibited a particular enzyme called COX-2.

I predicted three years before the scandal broke that it looked like a vascular catastrophe. I said it would probably inhibit the production of prostacyclin, which is the body's most important vascular lubricator. Lo and behold, it did. Look how many people were murdered as a result. I'm using the word "murder" because the drug company knew it was killing people. If it knew and kept it on the market, in my opinion, it's murder.

DR. KONDROT: Could you share with us some of the procedures and treatments you've learned over the years that you're incorporating now into your practice?

DR. ROWEN: My whole philosophy is based around three major causes of disease: improper nutrition or malnutrition, toxins, and stress. If you address these three, I think you can handle most everything else.

There are a couple of others. There's genetics, but that's minor. We're learning today that genetics are affected by your nutritional status and toxin load. There's exercise. There's whether you're getting sunlight, but that's a nutrient. There are a couple of others. There's injury.

I tend to look first at nutrition and toxins. Almost everybody I see is nutritionally deficient because they're eating the SAD, Standard American Diet, which is really poor. Our soils don't have minerals like they used to. The average American is eating processed food, further depleting the nutrients. They're eating cooked food, which further destroys the nutrients.

Then there are toxins. Almost everybody is dealing with heavy metals. There's mercury from dentists, lead that has been in the environment for years, chemicals, and pesticides.

DR. KONDROT: You're certainly a doctor who walks the talk. You probably have one of the healthiest diets I know. You're in excellent physical shape.

DR. ROWEN: Thanks. That's the first place I start. I'm an organic, raw food near-vegan. I eat limited amounts of dairy. Otherwise, I would be vegan. Almost everything I eat is uncooked, and I try to eat organic wherever possible. All of my numbers are absolutely ideal. In fact, I think I blew people away recently when I said that on a bad day, my blood pressure is 90 over 60.

DR. KONDROT: Every year, I hike with Dr. Rowen, and his stamina is amazing. His heart rate and blood pressure are well below normal. I think a big contributing factor to that is his very strict diet. My hat is off to you, Dr. Rowen.

DR. ROWEN: Thank you very much, Dr. Kondrot. You and I were on a hike just a couple of weeks ago in the High Sierra.

I think I scooted up a 1,000-foot, three-mile climb about ten minutes ahead of you and the other fellow.

DR. KONDROT: You did. I was huffing and puffing.

DR. KONDROT: Let's talk about the next topic you mentioned: detoxification. This is becoming a bigger problem in our society with heavy metal poisoning. How do you approach this, and what are some of the treatment options you offer your patients?

DR. ROWEN: Let's talk about the big two. The big two are mercury and lead. There are others. Cadmium is one. I was trained in intravenous chelation therapy a long time ago by the American College of Advancement in Medicine. IV chelation therapy is the gold standard for lead removal, no doubt. I used it for many years.

I'm gradually doing less IV chelation because I think I can accomplish the same with less expensive oral or rectal techniques. That way, patients can preserve their funds for other treatments that are definitely better given intravenously, like oxidation, which I will explain.

1. You can detox from mercury with supplements at home.

For mercury toxicity, I've never used intravenous or injectable treatments, preferring instead to use sulfur-bearing compounds like alpha lipoic acid or N-acetyl cysteine. I also use selenium, which binds and inactivates mercury on contact. I recommend vitamin C, sometimes chlorella. There are many people who use cilantro, but I haven't been part of that practice because I haven't seen evidence that I can sink my teeth into.

For mercury, my approach includes

1. 500 to 1,000 milligrams of alpha lipoic acid a day in divided doses;

2. 1,000 to 1,500 milligrams of NAC in divided doses;

3. Selenium as sodium selenite 200 micrograms;

4. maybe 2 to 3 grams of vitamin C and

5. maybe 15 small chlorella at night.

I've found, treating several thousand people in Alaska that this works for almost everybody in either three, six, or nine months. It took nine months to get my level down, but it worked, and it's not expensive.

DR. KONDROT: How do you diagnose lead or mercury poisoning?

DR. ROWEN: I give a capsule of DMPS for testing. Other doctors use DMPS for treatment. I never felt comfortable with it. I'm not saying it's wrong. I just use it for testing.

The patient wakes up in the morning, urinates, swallows a capsule, and then collects their urine for two hours or more. Then we measure the amount of heavy metals that come out. DMPS happens to grab lead, mercury, cadmium, arsenic, and others. Why? It's a sulfur-bearing compound, and the heavy metals seem to really like sulfur. They're attracted to sulfur.

DR. KONDROT: Once you collect the urine, you send it to a laboratory for analysis. How do you counsel the patient? Do you talk about dietary changes and look at certain environmental factors they might be exposed to?

DR. ROWEN: We have to get them eating organic and reduce their intake of toxins. As far as lead goes, I used to do a lot of IV chelation. I'm doing less now. Garry Gordon has been one of my long-term mentors. He has convinced me that you can address lead orally. His company has some products I really like. I used to use rectal EDTA suppositories when they were available. I have no doubt they work, and they're probably more cost effective than IV chelation.

IV chelation remains the best for lead. There's no doubt about it. If I think somebody is really suffering from lead, I then do intravenous chelation. If not, I'll take an oral route. I might take a rectal EDTA route. Generally, we see very nice results with heavy metal poisoning.

Arsenic is rather easy to treat. Selenium inactivates it. Sulfur-bearing compounds help get it out as well. Cadmium is a bit more difficult. I'd use intravenous chelation for that.

DR. KONDROT: I wonder if you could comment on the national study that was just completed, the TACT study that tried to assess chelation treatment. It has certainly caused a lot of excitement in alternative circles.

2. Chelation Therapy for heavy metals: now do it at home.

DR. ROWEN: I practiced in Alaska for 22 years, and a noted cardiologist called me a quack, wondering why I left a good career in emergency medicine to do quack chelation therapy. It turns out now that a study, Trial to Assess Chelation Therapy, was recently published in a major medical journal. The data was stunning.

The author presented his information to a crowd of cardiologists who expected to hear chelation debunked. It wasn't. It had excellent statistical significance. For diabetes, it was highly significant and very clear that anybody with vascular disease should consider intravenous chelation therapy.

DR. KONDROT: There are actually two reasons why individuals should consider chelation. One would be to improve their vascular status and the other to remove heavy metals, which are probably one of the greatest health hazards in our country.

DR. ROWEN: The heavy metals could be contributing to the vascular disease.

DR. KONDROT: I like your approach, moving from IV chelation to using rectal and oral, which in your opinion is just as effective and is much more economical. For people who need to tackle this problem, it is an investment. It takes 20 to 40 treatments (one to two treatments a week) before you begin to see a change.

DR. ROWEN: Doing oral chelation allows patients to do oxidation therapy. I love oxidation therapy. I've been doing it since 1986. This is a therapy, especially ozone therapy, which I have found to do more things for more people for more conditions than anything I've ever used in my life.

DR. KONDROT: That's a pretty powerful statement. When people hear of oxidative therapy and ozone, they think, "Isn't ozone a poisonous gas that's destroying the atmosphere? How can that possibly help improve my health?"

DR. ROWEN: Ozone in the atmosphere is a byproduct of automobile air pollution. You can't equate it with medical ozone, which is generated from medical-grade oxygen. It was found probably 80 or 90 years ago that when ozone gas of a low concentration was added to someone's blood, wonderful things happened. Their

immune system turned on. There was more oxygen delivery.

I'm an oxygen man. Do you remember that we were talking earlier about the three fundamental causes of disease? There's improper nutrition, toxins, and stress. Put that together with the fact a Nobel Prize winner, Otto Warburg, showed that you get cancer when the cells are consuming less oxygen or get less oxygen.

Oxygen is required for every cellular function. It's required to make energy. I want to get oxygen to the cells and get them stimulated to burn the oxygen and make energy so they can repair and do what they're supposed to do. If you can get them to make their own proteins and hormones, maybe you don't need to give hormones to people.

What does ozone do? I'll give you some examples. I can encourage your listeners to view my YouTube website. It is www. youtube.com/user/RobertRowenMD. I have treated patients who sometimes walk in the door crippled.

I video them before treatment, and they can barely get around the room. They're holding on to doors and walls just to walk. Then immediately after ozone gas is put into their knees, they're dancing around and swinging their hips in joy instantly.

People say to me, "That's impossible." Actually, it's not. Here's why. Where there's inflammation, there's poor circulation and a lack of oxygen. The inflammation itself is compromising blood supply.

It's swelling. There's less blood supply and less oxygen. It's a vicious cycle.

Ozone has been found to dramatically temper inflammation. It modulates cytokines and interferon so that the immune system is more balanced, whether you do it in blood or a joint. The presence of oxygen gives all those cells a lift to begin the repair process. Now, all of a sudden, they have the means to make the energy to repair themselves. That's why we see absolutely phenomenal results with shooting ozone into joints.

Its effect on the immune system is just one aspect of ozone. Ozone stimulates and balances cytokines. A researcher named Velio Bocci, in his book, describes ozone as the perfect cytokine inducer. Cytokines and interferons are the proteins and hormones that white blood cells use to talk to each other so that the immune system can go after the bad guy.

Another thing ozone does is enable red blood cells to actually deliver their oxygen at the capillary level. It also improves that rheology of blood. Rheology means the flow parameters. It keeps the red blood cells from sticking to each other and making a stack of coins in your capillaries. It keeps them repelling each other, so each cell runs through your capillary one at a time and doesn't clog it up.

3. Oxidation Therapies can cure even fatal diseases!

All of these basic properties combine to make ozone an extraordinarily powerful treatment. It's not a specific treatment. It's a nonspecific treatment that treats a wide variety of specific diseases. I've seen MRSA, methicillin-resistant staphylococcus aureus, clear up in one or two sessions. It's that fast.

Ozone is just one of three or more oxidation therapies. The others include ultraviolet blood irradiation therapy, intravenous hydrogen peroxide, and high-dose intravenous vitamin C therapy because vitamin C intravenous is not an antioxidant, as many people believe. It's actually a pro-oxidant because the vitamin C stimulates the production of hydrogen peroxide at the tissue level.

These are therapies we collectively call oxidation therapies, which I believe are among the most powerful healing therapies that humankind has ever known, and it doesn't involve chemicals.

DR. KONDROT: I know that you're a big advocate and teach oxidative courses to other physicians. In my experience, I agree with you. It's part of my practice treating people with chronic eye problems. It's hard to believe that in many states, oxidative treatments are illegal. Physicians cannot utilize these treatments.

DR. ROWEN: The reason why anything is illegal is because of the need to protect an inferior product? If your product doesn't work and it's inferior, the only way you can protect it is by having a monopoly on your inferior product. That's what has happened in this country today with pharma.

DR. KONDROT: I wonder if you could talk a little bit more about the delivery of ozone and these oxidative treatments. What can patients expect? If someone is suffering from a particular ailment, should they investigate oxidative treatment?

DR. ROWEN: They certainly could go online and type in "ozone therapy" or "ultraviolet blood irradiation therapy" and read about it. There's a lot of literature there, and there are a lot of articles that are posted worldwide at PubMed. That's free for anybody to see. They could try to locate somebody in their area who might do it.

There are two main therapies. One is ozone injection into joints or tissues. The other is ozone or ultraviolet treatment of blood where you take some blood out, expose it to ozone or ultraviolet, and re-infuse it into the patient.

The latter is a very powerful immune modulator stimulating circulation and fighting infection. It's an adjunctive treatment for cancer. By adjunctive, I mean it's a supportive treatment, not a primary treatment. It helps to detoxify the body. When you do all these things and you get your body to start burning oxygen, miracles can occur.

DR. KONDROT: It's hard to believe that such a simple treatment using a derivative of oxygen, ozone, which is O3, can produce these remarkable changes in the body. One thing we're both really excited with is the ability to self-administer ozone with rectal insufflation. I wonder if you could talk a little bit about that.

DR. ROWEN: Professor Silvia Menendez from Cuba has done remarkable research showing that rectal ozone can probably accomplish much or most of what intravenous ozone does. In my experience it does, but it works more slowly.

People can get ozone generators at home using medical-grade oxygen and administer it to themselves via rectal insufflation in the privacy of their home. This is absolutely legal to do because ozone machines can be used for water purification. You can adapt it in the privacy of your home for a rectal administration and see some stunning results. I like ozone. I use it on myself.

DR. KONDROT: I wanted to ask you about some of your favorite treatments that you're doing in your practice that are truly making a difference and making you excited about what you do.

DR. ROWEN: I would really suggest people go to that YouTube channel www.youtube.com/user/RobertRowenMD. There are a lot of videos where I'm being interviewed on YouTube, but please go to the channel so you can see patients.

What are we doing? We're doing a lot of what is called prolozone where we actually inject ozone gas into joints, and we're seeing marvelous results. People who were lame are recovering function and dancing around. It's simply remarkable.

There are people with chronic fatigue, fibromyalgia, and maybe even Lyme disease. There are a lot of people being told they have Lyme disease. Maybe they're infected, but their immune system is also failing.

I've treated symptoms like this since 1986 with ozone therapy. The results are generally remarkable. I'm not claiming I get 100%. No one does, but most people respond nicely.

Ultraviolet blood irradiation therapy has been around since the 1930s. There are scores of American papers. I wrote an article that is posted online. You can go to a small website, www.DocRowen.com, and get a link to my YouTube channel and to the article.

The article summarizes a lot of American research showing that 60 years ago, one or two treatments of ultraviolet blood irradiation was curing people of some of the worst infections you can imagine, the same diseases we can't treat today because of the failure of petrochemical antibiotics.

These are among the things I like. When somebody comes to me, I also look for other forms of toxicity in them, like root canals. I look in the mouth for mercury amalgams that could poison them. Root canals are basically dead teeth, and every tooth is connected to an acupuncture circuit. A dead tooth in an acupuncture circuit can knock out that whole circuit and cause dysfunction anywhere along the path of that meridian.

We've seen what some people would call miraculous recoveries. I don't call it miraculous. This is German medicine called neural therapy where you make a determination of scars or root canals causing disturbances in the body that can lead to dysfunction. You can sometimes get a result in an instant. When we take out an infected root canal — and I'm lucky to work with dentists who are willing to do this — the results can be stunning.

DR. KONDROT: You mentioned scars. How do scars interfere with energy conduction or these bio-meridians?

DR. ROWEN: The Germans believed that a scar produces an abhorrent, continuous, tiny electrical current into the nervous system that is sort of an irritant. It can reflex out at the same level or another level and cause a dysfunction.

I'll give you an example. Years ago in Alaska, I had a woman who had a lot of pain in her hip. Her orthopedic surgeon gave her an injection of steroids that didn't work. It caused atrophy at the site, which steroids do. I evaluated her and found a scar on her face and foot. I treated them both simply by injecting a local anesthetic into them, and her pain went away never to come back. It was a very simple injection. Yes, it's uncomfortable. Even injecting a local anesthetic into a scar is uncomfortable, but only during the time of the injection.

When it comes to root canals, I treated a woman with horrific back pain who needed help getting into the office. I said, "You don't have any good reason to have this pain. Your X-ray isn't bad, but they want to operate on you." She said yes. I asked if she has any root canals. She said she did. "Do you know where they are?" She did not. I did some muscle testing on her with what's called kinesiology, and I happened to find a tooth where she tested positive. She said, "I think that's a root canal." I treated it. Nothing happened to her pain. I tested each additional tooth until I found a second one. Then I treated that tooth. Lo and behold, she jumped off the table, did a jig, and said, "What did you do?" I said, "Your pain is probably going to come back. I want that tooth X-rayed."

She had a dentist X-ray it. They found a hidden abscess at the apex of the tooth and took it out. Her pain went away. When she finally passed away years later, she did not have back pain.

DR. KONDROT: That's an amazing story. Most people don't look at their dental health as a contributing factor to chronic disease or severe pain.

DR. ROWEN: That's true. The body is an integrated whole. A disturbance in one part of the body can potentially affect a totally different part of the body. You're not going to be treating that simply by taking a petrochemical pain suppressant. You need to see if you can find the actual cause.

DR. KONDROT: I know you also like to treat with high doses of vitamin C. I wonder if you could comment on high doses of vitamin C intravenously.

DR. ROWEN: Vitamin C was found by Dr. Klenner many years ago to cure polio and infections. He was scoffed at and laughed at until the National Institute of Health started doing research in the last six years. They have found that when you take vitamin C, ascorbic acid, in levels achievable only intravenously, your tissues actually produce hydrogen peroxide. This peroxide can move into cells, potentially knocking out cancer cells and stimulating the immune system because hydrogen peroxide is a messenger. Sadly, it's not being used by conventional medicine.

DR. KONDROT: Could you give us a closing comment, Dr. Rowen? It was certainly a pleasure having you on the show.

DR. ROWEN: My goal is to try to keep you out of my office. Please eat right. Don't eat the standard American diet. If 70% to 80% of what you eat is alive and chemical free when it goes into your mouth, you'll go a long way to improving your health. Try to reduce stress. Get exercise. Detoxify with saunas and sweats for organic chemicals and use some form of chelation or nutritional therapy for heavy metals. Oxidation therapy could do a lot for the rest for you. At least, it does in my experience.

....

ROBERT ROWEN, MD
Santa Rosa California
http://www.doctorrowen.com/
(707)578-7787

Charles Schwengel, DO, DO(H)

MESA, ARIZONA

November 3, 2013

1. **You do not need to have cancer treatment tomorrow or die. The first step is to relax.**

2. **Nature has provided a recovery mechanism, and it has been there since the beginning of time.**

3. **We don't need chemotherapies, surgeries, and radiation. We don't need to fight cancers. We need to work with nature.**

DR. KONDROT: Today my guest is Charles Schwengel, a member of the Arizona Homeopathic and Integrative Medical Association. He is very active in the Arizona integrative medical community and is doing groundbreaking research in nutritional treatment for cancer. I thought we could start with some background information on how you got interested in medicine and how you made the transition to embracing alternative therapies.

DR. SCHWENGEL: I've thought in terms of what we call alternative today from the very beginning. That's how I got interested in medicine. It incorporates ways of doing treatments for the body and keeping healthy that are aligned with nature. That was my original inspiration, and that has never wavered. Of course, I've found over the years what that really means and how expansive that is. It's a huge field.

DR. KONDROT: It's probably one of the reasons you became a doctor of osteopathic medicine.

DR. SCHWENGEL: I like the hands-on treatment we can do. You learn how to work with the structure of the body, like the muscles and joints, and realign and repair injuries and damage, and take away pain. Of course, that leads into nutrition, which leads into homeopathy and the whole field. Here we are. Today, we call it alternative and integrative.

DR. KONDROT: Let's move right into your major interest. You're actively involved in helping people who are suffering from cancer who have had traditional chemotherapy and or radiation and are suffering from a lot of the side effects. Not only are you helping folks recover, but you're also helping them in their cancer treatment. What should patients be aware of in their options for cancer treatment? Often, traditional doctors really don't tell them what their options are.

DR. SCHWENGEL: Absolutely so. Let's begin with a little bit of background. I practiced natural medicine and homeopathic therapies for a wide variety of general medical conditions and stayed away from cancer for quite a while. Like most doctors, when I was a student in school, and even in practice, we were sort of trained to be afraid. You're afraid of the diagnosis. You're afraid to talk to patients. You're afraid of the therapies, and you're afraid of final outcomes.

In a subconscious way, I did realize that. Then a friend of mine said something about low-dose chemotherapy. I looked

into that and learned how that works. You can do treatments that actually use chemotherapy medications but don't have the side effects. I found out it's helpful to do that. You get a better quality of life, although ultimately the outcomes are about the same. Still, the patient's quality of life is improved. I was impressed with that. Then, I realized that I have an entire protocol and a lot of resources in terms of nutritional and homeopathic things to help support, strengthen, and cleanse the body throughout this entire process.

Today, we're reaching out to people like you just described, those who are dealing with cancer as well as people who have already had treatments and are dealing with some of those side effects. As you well know, the side effects from the therapies themselves can be severe. You can get sick and really threaten your health because of the treatment alone, let alone the original cancer.

People aren't given choices. All too often, you might get diagnosed today and then tomorrow you're supposed to start some form of chemotherapy, surgery, or radiation therapy without giving any thought as to why this cancer has developed and if there are any other options to deal with it.

A great many people are looking for options. They just don't know where to go. Kudos to you, Dr. Kondrot, for producing a book like this and making it available for people who want another source of reliable information.

DR. KONDROT: Let me ask you this. Let's say someone is diagnosed with cancer. The first thing that occurs is there is a lot of fear. The doctor will tell you that unless you have chemotherapy or surgery, you're going to die. You're put into that fear state, which certainly doesn't help your body heal. If you're not in a balanced autonomic state, as you and I well know, the body doesn't heal. What do you advise patients to do? In traditional medicine, they talk about all the quacks out there and people going to Mexico expecting a cure but they die. They paint a very horrible picture. How can a patient be objective?

DR. SCHWENGEL: The first thing in being objective and overcoming the fear is to realize this. What we call cancers are the tumors that grow on the body and become noticed at some point because of some kind of test or symptom, like a mammogram or prostate test or some kind of lump or bump that develops. Then you go to the doctor and they check it out, take some pictures, or do a biopsy, and, finally, they call it cancer.

1. You do not need to have cancer treatment tomorrow or die. The first step is to relax.

Those things are transformations inside the body. They are transformations of some part of your natural self and your natural organs and tissues. When you think about that for a minute, we have natural bodies. Why does nature allow those transformations to happen? Then it becomes a short step to realize that nature always has a reason and purpose for making the changes that nature does. Nature is never random, so there has to be a reason.

Let's think about what the reason might be and understand that this is not a crisis or emergency. You do not need to have treatment tomorrow or else die. That's what's put into most people's heads, so the first step is to relax. You nailed it on the head just a moment ago. You said autonomic nerves. What that really means is that most people are scared. They're put into, because of fear, a state of sympathetic drive.

Sympathetic energy is the kind of energy you have during the day. You have to get up, go, do things, and get things done. You have a sympathetic drive in the body. Cancers grow during sympathetic drive. Fear stimulates that sympathetic drive. The other side of the coin is rest, which happens at the end of the day. You go to bed. Now it's nighttime, and your body will heal. That's parasympathetic. To be able to relax and let go of the fear will stimulate that healing phase of the parasympathetic energies. That's the biggest part of the problem. People are unknowingly or unwillingly put into a state of fear which drives their sympathetic energy which causes the cancers to grow more.

DR. KONDROT: I like your analogy that we're natural bodies, and we need to look to nature. I was thinking of a homeopathic principle that states that the body has wisdom. Whenever you develop a disease, even if it's cancer, there is a reason. The body needs that cancer to maintain homeostasis or balance. Can you talk about the laws of nature when it comes to organs and cancer? From what you say, this really isn't some type of random event or toss of the dice.

DR. SCHWENGEL: That's exactly true. When you look at the natural world, realize there's always a purpose in everything that happens. Everything you see has a reason and a purpose. Nothing happens at random. Sometimes something will look random, but when you examine it and dig deeper, it really isn't. There's a reason and a purpose, and there are results in things that happen in nature.

Of course, we're born in and live in natural bodies, so what happens in the body also has natural reason and natural purpose. When it comes to the transformation of tissues in the organs that develop lumps and bumps that we eventually diagnose and call cancer, there is a natural reason and purpose for that. It's not random, and it's not always because of toxicity, inherence, or other causes that people attribute to it.

There is a mind to body connection, and that's one of the core points we need to discuss. It's how what happens in the mind precedes what happens in the body. To say that a different way and with more

depth, let us discuss stress. We live with stress all the time. It requires stress to get up and function throughout the day and solve problems. You have a stress, solve the problem, and feel good about that, and life goes on.

When you have a kind of stress that is much bigger than your ability to address or cope, something that is severe with no solution in sight, that's when the mind begins to cause the body to transform in a way that develops tumors. I will give some more concrete examples later that illustrate why that happens.

For the moment, it's important to think of it in a different way. What I'm inviting patients to do is think about what they're doing when it comes to cancer and cancer treatments.

If we could control nature with therapies, chemotherapy, radiation, or surgery, I'd be all for it, but we can't. I don't know any way that we can control nature. What we can do is support the body and enhance, facilitate, and encourage it, but we can't control it.

One of the best things I think we can do is talk to the mind so that the mind can heal the body. As we just said, the mind becomes altered due to the stress that precedes what happens to the body.

Homeopathic medicine has a unique ability because it is information medicine. It's like a language, and we can use that language to give messages to the mind. The messages really have to do with easing the kind of stress that's going on.

DR. KONDROT: I like that approach. Being an alternative eye doctor, I have always thought there is an emotional component to eye disease that may be hidden or buried. The patient may not be aware of it, but it usually is there. You're right about homeopathy. Homeopathy is probably one of the most elegant ways of combining the emotional symptoms with the physical symptoms.

If you have a particular tumor and you're looking at the characteristics of that tumor, you're also looking at certain emotional characteristics. If it's the right remedy, you're going to be matching both the emotional and physical symptoms to get a remarkable change in the person. Unfortunately, most traditional Western doctors don't take that approach. They look at the tumor as something evil, and something we need to destroy.

DR. SCHWENGEL: I understand. Hats off to traditional doctors because they're trying to do their best, and their hearts are in the right place. They're doing what they know to be the standard of medical care, and they are consistent with their training. You can't fault them for that. The problem lies much deeper in that it's not the individual doctors; it's the system that doesn't think about why a tumor has appeared or realize they have to work with nature.

Of course, we all think about fight. Every time you get diagnosed or hear about somebody with a serious diagnosis, the next word out of your mouth is "fight." You hear that you have to fight cancer everywhere you look. It's all over the radio shows, television, and media. There is a lot of research and fundraising that goes on about the fight against cancer.

Let's apply that concept to what we just talked about. If we live in natural bodies and we're obeying the laws of nature at a conscious level or not, if we're going to *fight* cancer, which is transformations in our body, then that is exactly the same thing as fighting against nature. I can't think of a good example of a person picking a fight with nature and winning. I don't know that we should be fighting nature. Cancer is not something to fight. It is something to be overcome, of course, and to be healed from.

The way I like to look at it and the way we talk about it is that healing is not fighting. There is nothing healing about fight, and there is no fight in healing. It goes both ways. Healing involves reducing and finding ways to remove and resolve the stress. It is detoxification. It is nutritional replenishment and all the related support. We cannot control healing. We can facilitate, encourage, and support it, but we can't control it.

I think most of the Western medicine approach, the conventional thing with chemotherapy, radiation, and surgery, is an effort to control the ultimate result of a long-term natural process. They're doing what they think is best, but in actuality, it's really not the right thing to do. The right thing to do is healing, and it has to start from inside. Healing has to come from the inside out, and it has to rest with each person, not with the doctor.

An extension of that comment is when people ask, "What is your success rate?" My answer is, "I don't have a success rate." The success comes from inside each person. How willing is each person to let go of his or her stress, identify it, participate in the program, and let healing happen from the inside out in a very natural way instead of trying to fight in a very unnatural way?

DR. KONDROT: Please describe how you approach a patient. How is your evaluation different from more conventional doctors? What do you look for?

DR. SCHWENGEL: In terms of integrative medicine, the evaluations I do are the standard kind of thing. I'm very interested in physical exams, blood tests, and imaging. Imaging means things like X-rays, PET scans, and MRIs. These kinds of diagnostics are important because you need to know where you are when you start. If you're going to start a journey, even a journey of healing, you need to know where you are so you can determine how far you're making progress along the way to recovery.

2. Nature has provided a recovery mechanism, and it has been there since the beginning of time.

When it comes to therapy, that's a whole different issue. Nature has provided a recovery mechanism, and it has been there since the beginning of time. We can take advantage of it. It is right at our fingertips. This is one of the most amazing things I have ever learned. Let me share it with you now. We're born with natural bodies, and we live with natural laws. Nature knows. Those important words are something people need to remember. Nature knows. Nature knows in advance, as it were, when we're going to have stresses in life and that our mind will cause the body to transform in such a way that it grows tumors that become what we call cancers.

Wouldn't you know that nature has already provided a means to reverse and recover from that process? It's been there since the beginning of time. It's in our foods and herbs and things we eat that are grown by nature.

A couple of researchers from a university in Victoria, Canada, published a little book about how cancer cells have an enzyme inside them. In some of our natural food components, there's a class of products that will stimulate the enzyme inside the cancer cells to go through what's called a programmed cell death.

The medical word for that is apoptosis. It's a programmed cell death which means when you eat the right foods, the nutrients in the herbs and foods get into the cancer cells, activate this enzyme, and then the cancer cell goes through a self-destruction process. It breaks down into component parts, and all those parts are recycled.

3. We don't need chemotherapies, surgeries, and radiation. We don't need to fight cancers. We need to work with nature.

This is a very natural process, and the process is stimulated by the right foods. All we have to do is eat and consume the right foods and herbs in sufficient quantity to stimulate that natural programmed cell death process. That is absolutely the best way to recover from cancers and tumors.

I don't believe we need to have chemotherapies, surgeries, and radiation. We don't need to fight cancers. We need to work with nature and cooperate with what nature has already provided us.

There has been a great deal of research about different kinds of herb products and why they do this. This is my approach. I have a product line I use that are natural herbs, organic, raw products that are drawn from around the world and processed in ways to protect their natural goodness.

They are not preserved, cooked, or harmed in any way that their natural food values are compromised. These foods are protected and processed in a way that maintains their natural goodness. They're easy to take, so I have a wide variety of products to use. I put together packages of pills for each patient.

When somebody comes to us, we do an evaluation. I'm interested in all the blood testing, imaging, and the things we have to do to establish the diagnosis. Then instead of doing chemotherapy, we'll start this nutrition approach. Now you have the natural herbs that are helping the body become healthier and causing the cancer cells to kill themselves all at the same time. What a powerful combination that is.

DR. KONDROT: I think Hippocrates said that food is our best medicine. You're going back to the ancient roots when people did treat disease by changing their diet and eating the right foods.

DR. SCHWENGEL: That's exactly right. How wise he was to say that. To depend on nature makes so much sense. If we live in natural bodies, use natural processes for our natural health.

There's always a time and place for conventional medicine and the things it does. I'm certainly glad it's there. On the other hand, I wouldn't encourage everybody to think medicine has all the answers because it does not. When it comes to something as pervasive and as problematic as cancer, you need to think about natural products. That's the option.

DR. KONDROT: That's my main approach. When someone comes to me with a chronic eye problem, the first thing I do is clean up his or her diet.

DR. SCHWENGEL: I've had a number of patients in my office who have gone to you just for that problem. They've been very pleased with their results.

DR. KONDROT: Are your nutritional products specific for the type of cancer or the person? How are these products formulated?

DR. SCHWENGEL: That's a very good question. When you talk about herbal products, it's pretty easy to get too much. It's like anything else. There's a therapeutic level and an overdose. We don't want to overdose on the herbs, so I use a small amount of a wide variety so you don't get too much of anything.

I have about 180 different herbs that are combined in the packages we use. The herbal foundation is the same for everybody. However, there is also a component that guides the healing toward the specific tissue. A good word for that is micro RNAs. RNA stands for ribonucleic acid, which is the counterpart to DNA, which is what causes our cells to grow the way they do. To help heal the cells in the DNA, we can use the micro RNAs from specific sources to help target the herbal concentrates to the organs and tissues you want to heal.

For example, we have the micro RNAs, like the herbal products for breast, liver, prostate, lung, or whatever the condition or body part is. The herbal foundation is pretty much the same, but the focus of it has to do with these little RNAs. That is what we can use to focus the healing and stimulate that process in just about any body part you care to focus on.

DR. KONDROT: When someone is on your program, is it also necessary to begin detoxification? Some doctors feel strongly about removing heavy metals which may contribute to the disease. What's your opinion on that?

DR. SCHWENGEL: There is so much in the environment that we take for granted, not realizing how toxic it is. Detoxification is built into our whole program, partly with the homeopathic formulas I use and partly with the natural herbs. Natural herbs have a little-known but well-documented effect of detoxifying from heavy metals. I have research articles that show how well they take out mercury, lead, aluminum, and other things we have problems with. Then, of course, there is tissue cleansing, liver cleansing, and the digestive system. The detoxification process is already built into the program.

DR. KONDROT: When someone goes on your program, how long does it typically take? Do you monitor the progression of the tumor? What's your end point for success?

DR. SCHWENGEL: The tumors and the cancers are something where we like to think in terms of cure. Many of us know of somebody who has gotten over his or her cancer. The time that it takes depends on each person because of that mind/body connection. The duration of the tumors is actually connected to how deeply it is in your mind and how intense it is. That is not something physical, and we can't control that. Having said that, most people respond pretty well in four to six months, although it's probably going to be a year or two of maintenance. Of course, we don't talk about cure until you're five years in remission.

DR. KONDROT: What about the individual who wants to have chemotherapy and use this as an adjunctive treatment?

DR. SCHWENGEL: I'll tell you something else about options in Western medicine. They tell people who are having chemotherapy not to take antioxidants, vitamin C, or the kind of vitamins that most of us alternative and integrative doctors would recommend because they're afraid it will interfere with the therapeutic value of the chemotherapy. The actual truth is exactly the opposite. There is a lot of research that shows that when you take antioxidants and extra vitamin C, it actually enhances the therapeutic effect of chemotherapy medications, and it decreases the side effects. People are better protected from the side effects, and they get better results from the chemotherapy.

For those people who are going to do the chemotherapy, it's important that they look into this for themselves and find somebody qualified who has looked into it to give this kind of information.

DR. KONDROT: Unfortunately, most patients are put into a fear state and don't take any vitamins or nutritional supplements because they are afraid that it will interfere with their treatment.

DR. SCHWENGEL: Probably the most exciting thing I've ever encountered is why it is that we develop tumors in the first place. For any body part, there is going to be a story behind it. I call that a plot. The plot is pretty much the same for all people, although the storyline and the details belonging to each person are as unique as they are. The plot behind it is the same.

Let's talk about some of the more common kinds of cancers. Breast cancer is the biggest one for women. When they develop breast cancer, women are concerned about hereditary consider-ations and genetics, or they're concerned about toxicities. They overlook the fact that each body organ has a purpose and an emotional connection to it. The mind/body connection is just as important in cancer as it is in any other kind of illness.

When you think of it that way, you realize that a woman's breast is designed for nurturing. Whom does the woman nurture? She nurtures children, of course. The most likely thing when a woman develops a breast tumor is that she has some kind of nurturing stress with her children. I've seen that so many times.

Here's a more interesting part. A right-handed woman will develop the tumor on her left side first, and it's the other way around for a left-handed woman. That is because of the way nature has developed and the way we handle things. When a right-handed woman is nursing her baby, she'll hold it in her left arm and nurse it from the left breast so that her dominant hand, her right hand, is available to care for, pamper, and nurture the baby. In a left-handed woman, it's the other way around. She'll be nursing on the right side. When a mother has some kind of stress with the offspring and begins to develop tumors, you look on the side first that's opposite her dominant side.

Let's talk about the kinds of stresses that happen. Things I have seen so many times are stresses of the nurturing, like, "How can I protect my child?" or "My child is in trouble and needs help," or something like that. It's the sort of situation that can develop suddenly and unexpectedly, but mostly it has no end in sight. There are a lot of forces on the planet, but I don't know of a force much stronger than that of a mother's protection of her child. I think that's true in a great many species. Mammals all around the planet think that way. When a mother thinks her child is in trouble or needs protection and she can't protect it, that's when this kind of thing begins to happen.

There are other kinds of examples. Let's talk about liver cancer and even the digestive. Almost always, when tumors develop in the digestive system, there will be anger. It's anger toward someone, some situation or even toward self, specifically when we talk about the pancreas.

So many people have pancreas cancer. They know it's a fast-growing, difficult thing. The pancreas is actually connected to a concept of anger toward family, and

sometimes family is the person themselves. It can also be some family member.

When I look at somebody's diagnosis, right away I know what the plot is. Most of us in integrative medicine are aware of this. There are ways of asking the mind, through the body, questions. We can do muscle testing or computerized testing called electrodermal screening or EAV. I use that kind of testing to evaluate the nature of the stress.

I don't know about you, but I prefer not to say words like "always" and "never" when I'm talking to patients. I think it's medically irresponsible, but I'll tell you my experience. I have had the opportunity to test this kind of theory over 2,000 times, and not once have I found an exception to it. Every single time, the story fits. When I have somebody with a diagnosis and I know where it is, I can tell him or her why it's there. The muscle testing or this electrodermal testing supports that. I don't know of any other kind of medical treatment that has that kind of record.

DR. KONDROT: Do you think that when the patient is aware of this conflict, they need some type of support in dealing with what comes to the surface? Does that help in the healing of the tumor?

DR. SCHWENGEL: That depends on each person, and very often they do. Many times, the patient understands and knows what the nature of the conflict is. That's exactly the right word. We call it biological conflict when the stresses become sufficient to create changes in the body. Many people know what it is and acknowledge it. Other times it's kind of a surprise, and they don't know; yet, the story fits. They say, "Now that you say it, this is true."

I always recommend that they talk to somebody they can trust to help heal that particular part of the mind/body relationship if it is with the person themselves. Maybe it's with a parent and the parent has passed on, or they really can't talk to them anymore. They can talk to a friend, minister, or counselor. Sometimes a professional counselor will help. That's a variable according to each person's needs. Not everybody needs that.

When you unlock the door where the skeletons in the closet are hidden, you let the skeletons out, and you have to deal with it. That is the scariest and sometimes the most difficult part about the healing process. It isn't the therapies. It's letting go of hanging onto the stress. That's a difficult thing for some people.

DR. KONDROT: How do you help patients deal with letting go of the stress and letting the skeletons come out of the closet? Are there certain techniques you use?

DR. SCHWENGEL: This connects the whole circle. We come back to homeopathy again. Nature provides energy in our foods and herbs. Homeopathic medicines can do that. We well know that many healing experiences have to do with unlocking a barrier to a relationship with parents, for example, or with unlocking fears about various kinds of things, like fires, sharp objects, or many other things. It's easy to create a homeopathic formula that helps ease the process of opening the door and dealing with whatever comes up.

DR. KONDROT: Homeopathy can act as a powerful catalyst to get the whole system moving in the right direction. How can people contact you?

DR. SCHWENGEL: I'd like to talk to people before they make an appointment or make plans to come see me. They have to visit me once to get this set up. After that, I can send them the products and keep a supply going for quite a long time. They stay at home and continue their life, work, and family life.

....

CHARLES SCHWENGEL DO, DO(H)
Mesa, Arizona
(480)668-1448
www.RhythmOfLife.com

Frank Shallenberger, MD, MD(H), ABAAM

CARSON CITY, NEVADA

Interviewed October 20, 2013

1. Antioxidants won't make you live longer; for that, you need oxidative therapy.

2. A doctor who is not yet offering ozone therapy to his patients is practicing substandard medicine.

3. Ozone cures pain — any pain.

DR. KONDROT: I would like to introduce my good friend, Dr. Frank Shallenberger, who is a leading authority on ozone treatment. He holds a phenomenal educational course on ozone treatment and is responsible for testing and certifying doctors to become members of the American Academy of Ozone Therapy. Dr. Shallenberger, I wonder if you could share how you got started in alternative treatments and how you developed an interest in oxidative treatment and ozone.

DR. SHALLENBERGER: It started back in the early '80s. I was really interested in alternative medicine at the time. I went to hear a lecture by Charlie Farr. Charlie was a PhD in chemistry and a medical doctor. Charlie was infusing hydrogen peroxide into patients intravenously, and they were getting better.

At the time, that was shocking because the early '80s was a time when everybody started to hear about how bad oxidants were supposed to be and how supposedly good antioxidants were. Here's Charlie saying, "I'm giving my patient an oxidant, and he's getting better." That flew in the face of what everybody else thought was right and intelligent. I was immediately intrigued. Charlie really did his homework. He investigated the therapy and gave a great lecture. That's when I learned something very interesting, which is that oxidants have their role in human metabolism, and they're not necessarily bad. After that, I began to use hydrogen peroxide with my patients. I infused it intravenously. Just like Charlie said, a lot of people got better.

DR. KONDROT: That's probably a little disturbing to some people. We've been hearing that you need antioxidants to keep your body healthy. Now you're saying that giving an oxidative agent like hydrogen peroxide can be beneficial. Maybe you could explain why that is so.

DR. SHALLENBERGER: There are industries making millions from promoting the idea that if you take antioxidant nutrients in larger doses than you get from your nutrition — if you take a lot of antioxidant vitamins, for example — you're going to live longer, and you're not going to get sick.

1. Antioxidants won't make you live longer; for that, you need oxidative therapy.

What the literature shows us is that that's just not true. There are absolutely no studies, animal or human, that demonstrate that taking antioxidants in the form of vitamins and extra supplements can make you live any longer or prevent any diseases. It just doesn't happen; yet, that's what most people think.

What we do know now is that the exact opposite is true. What makes you sick is a lack of oxidation, which is what antioxidants oppose. It's hard getting the word out because we have this whole commercial industry out there that wants to convince everybody that taking antioxidant pills is the way to go. Forget the antioxidant pills. You get plenty of antioxidants if your diet is good. Start doing therapies that promote oxidation. Studies show that oxidation is what promotes longevity and prevents disease. In fact, oxidation can be used to cure people of the diseases they have.

Let me put it this way. Most people have probably heard that exercise, when properly done, prevents just about every disease there is. Recently, there was a study of patients who have cancer. In this particular study, some of them got chemotherapy. The others did not get chemotherapy and just got exercise. They did better than the ones who got chemotherapy. We all know that exercise is a very powerful preventer of disease. Exercise is an example of oxidation therapy.

2. A doctor who is not yet offering ozone therapy to his patients is practicing substandard medicine.

DR. KONDROT: You have said that if any doctor is not doing oxidative or ozone treatments, they need to learn that they're actually doing their patients a disservice. Could you clarify that or expand on that comment?

DR. SHALLENBERGER: It's a radical thing

to say that if a doctor isn't offering a particular therapy to his patient then he's doing him a disservice, but I have to say this is true for ozone therapy.

Ozone therapy takes away pain. If it only did that, what doctor in his right mind would want to deprive his patient of something that takes away pain? Of all the things that we as doctors do, maybe the most wonderful and most beautiful is to remove patients' pain. Ozone is absolutely astounding for that. I feel it's okay to make that comment.

Ozone does a lot of other things. It can cure chronic hepatitis C and common chronic viral illnesses, from herpes to shingles to hepatitis B to influenza.

You have a therapy at your fingertips that costs pennies; it's absolutely safe, and you don't need to have informed consent. We have to get this out. I'm sure if doctors really understood how great this was, they'd be flocking to learn about it.

DR. KONDROT: I just returned from the World Ozone Congress in Rome, Italy. There were 27 nations represented at this congress and over 95 presentations were delivered. It was a phenomenal meeting. It's amazing how accepted ozone therapy is in many European countries; yet, here in the United States, the FDA has taken the position that ozone is dangerous. It's shocking.

I agree with you 100%. I've been doing ozone treatments for eye patients for the last ten years. It's such an important treatment and can actually help reverse disease. Not only can it help reverse eye disease, but it improves the general health of the patient. I always hate to say something is a general cure-all, but I think with ozone and oxidative treatments you can say that because it is essentially anti-aging. It reverses the aging process. When you do get disease, it's due to aging. Maybe you can talk a little more about the mechanism, how it works, and how it helps treat disease.

DR. SHALLENBERGER: We do know a lot about the mechanism. It has to do directly with this process called oxidation. For many, that's going to be a difficult concept to get. If I simplify it, I would say that oxidation is the process by which oxygen is converted into the energy that keeps us alive. It is the most fundamental process that goes on in the body. Virtually half the activity of every single cell in your body is involved in oxidation. You can't remain alive for more than two or three minutes without oxidation.

Most people think that if they're breathing and taking in oxygen, everything is good. I'd venture to say most doctors think that. If you're taking in oxygen, then oxygen is not a problem. All you have to do is get it in your body. This is not true. There's a mechanism by which we process that oxygen. Over time, that mechanism fails. One of the things that causes it to fail is getting older. Other things are things you talk about all the time, like toxicity, nutritional deficiency, stress, hormonal deficiencies, and all these kinds of things that also decrease the body's ability to process the oxygen.

Here's the thing. If you're taking in a lot of oxygen but you can only process 40% of it, you might as well only be taking in 40% as much oxygen. You're not getting anything out of it.

That's the process of oxidation. What's remarkable is that ozone stimulates that. If people will just get that through their heads, "Ozone therapy is going to help my body use its oxygen better," then they can realize what a dramatic therapy this is.

DR. KONDROT: That's the way I explain the mechanism to some of my patients. Everybody understands oxygen saturation. You're breathing oxygen. It's in your arterial circulation. It's healthy for you. You need oxygen, but you don't really know how your cells are utilizing that oxygen.

That's the amazing thing about ozone and oxidative treatments. They improve the oxygen utilization. When that happens, you can reverse the aging process and dramatically stimulate the body to heal. I think most people understand that. You and I have to convince the physicians and medical doctors to begin to look at this.

In the meeting in Europe, 27 nations were represented and there were 95 amazing papers presented, showing all aspects of the benefits of ozone. Here in the United States, what are we going to do? I know you are helping spread the word through your course, which is phe-

nomenal. I'm going to be taking it again for the second time. There is so much material.

DR. SHALLENBERGER: The thing doctors have to realize is that this is something that fits into everything they're already doing. If they're talking to their patients about detoxification, getting a better diet, supplementing with various nutrients and such, exercise, or no matter what they're talking to their patients about, they're going to get better results if they add this principle of oxidation.

DR. KONDROT: At the World Meeting, there were a couple of interesting papers that showed that when you add oxidative treatments to a standard care, the results improve dramatically. Although you could look at it as replacing a lot of standard treatments, I think it could be also a good adjunctive treatment.

DR. SHALLENBERGER: For example, there are infections. Studies have shown that if you have an infection and you treat it with an antibiotic, you're going to cure a certain percentage of the infection. If to that antibiotic you also add ozone therapy, you increase the efficacy of curing the infection by 20% or 30% just by adding that.

DR. KONDROT: Dr. Shallenberger, I wonder if you can talk a little bit about the ways of administering oxidative treatments. They are certainly varied. Maybe you can go into some specialized techniques that you have found have really benefited patients.

DR. SHALLENBERGER: That's one of the beauties. Earlier on, I talked about hydrogen peroxide therapy, which is a great therapy. The thing about that is it's very limited. You can only use it in certain ways.

With ozone therapy, it seems that there are no limits to it at all. You can apply ozone to virtually any body cavity or any part of the body. You can add it to the blood. You can give it as an enema into the colon. You can put it in the bladder, down the stomach, or through the skin in the form of a sauna. We do all of that in my clinic.

We can treat blood directly with ozone. We can inject ozone into various areas of the body. We can put it in joints to help the joints heal. If the patient is having pain in literally any part of his body, we can just inject ozone into that part of the body. The applicability is astounding.

If I am seeing 20 patients in a given day, I'm probably going to use ozone on 15 of them. The usefulness in so many different varieties of illnesses and problems that people have is astounding when it comes to this particular molecule.

That shouldn't be too shocking because we're talking about oxygen. I don't know if people appreciate the fact that ozone is an extra excitable molecule of oxygen. If I were to treat their blood with oxygen, I would get a good result. If I were to treat their blood with ozone, I would get the same result I did with the oxygen, only dramatically intensified.

DR. KONDROT: We've been hearing about hyperbaric oxygen and people going into oxygen chambers to help rejuvenate and reverse different pathological conditions. What you're saying is that the ozone molecule has a much more powerful effect. It gives a better kick than oxygen under concentration.

DR. SHALLENBERGER: Yes, it does. Hyperbaric oxygen's job is to deliver more oxygen to an area. The problem with people most of the time is not that they don't have enough oxygen in the area. The problem is that they have a lot of oxygen to the area. They just can't use it. Hyperbaric doesn't really address that issue; ozone therapy does. Actually, you can use the two together.

DR. KONDROT: You make a really good point. The key with oxidative treatments is that they're helping to improve oxygen utilization. That's what the body needs to regenerate and get healthy.

Could you talk a little more in detail about the different methods of administration? Two methods that are in popular use are IV and rectal. What are your favorites? Which ones do you feel work more effectively?

DR. SHALLENBERGER: The first thing that comes to my mind is treating the bladder.

There's a condition of the bladder called chronic interstitial cystitis, which is similar to a chronic bladder infection. It's a terrible disorder. A lot of women have it. A few men have it, but it's mostly a female thing. There are no known conventional treatments for it. If you inject ozone into a woman's bladder, you flat-out cure this condition virtually 100% of the time, even if it's been there for 20 years. That, in itself, is a dramatic situation. When I see such a patient, one of the first things that occurs to me is being able to treat a bladder with such a severe problem easily, safely, and inexpensively, and have it result in a cure. We do it that way, of course.

Another treatment that I think is overlooked by a lot of practitioners throughout the world is starting to get more recognition now. It is treating with ozone through the skin. You can put patients into a chamber, kind of like a sauna, and apply ozone gas to the skin. It gets absorbed through the skin and creates a number of very fascinating healing effects by that modality.

Many of us integrative doctors have used it through the blood where we draw some blood out, treat the blood with the ozone, and then re-infuse the treated blood back in. That requires a needle, a doctor's office, and things like that. Something like an ozone sauna is very dramatic in what it can do, so we're learning more about that.

If you were to come to my office with a chronic disease, odds are pretty good you're going to get ozone in every single one of the forms I've mentioned to you. The more different ways you can apply this to the human body, the better that body heals.

DR. KONDROT: There were a couple of papers presented in Italy about using different methods of ozone, like major arterial therapy where it's mixed with the blood, injected in the particular tissue, or used in a sauna preparation. There was a lot of interest in saunas. The saunas are increasing in popularity. I want you to talk a little bit about rectal insufflation. More people are becoming interested in that as an effective way of administering ozone without the need for an IV.

DR. SHALLENBERGER: I've very excited about this. I'm of the opinion that every single person ought to have their own ozone generator and be able to administer ozone to themselves via the rectum. We've known for a long time that if you put medicines into the rectum, whether it's penicillin or any other kind of medicine, they get absorbed into the bloodstream almost as quickly as if you actually injected it. Ozone works this way.

What's interesting about that method is that it's completely safe and easy. Patients can do it to themselves. It's my preferred treatment for my own personal use. A couple of times a week, I'll give myself a treatment this way. I'd rather do it that way than have a needle stuck into me. It works every bit as well. This is something you can do at home.

DR. KONDROT: This is the type of treatment where you can empower patients. They can do the treatment daily or every other day to tackle a chronic disease or a serious medical problem. Dr. Shallenberger, what are the uses of ozone that really get you excited or that really amaze you every time you do it?

DR. SHALLENBERGER: I'm glad you asked that. When patients come in to see me, they may have chronic pain, for example, chronic back pain. So many people have it. They take drugs for it and get surgery for it. Some people suffer dramatically due to their back pain.

Doctors have nothing to offer them except surgery, which some of them have already had, and it just made them worse or didn't help. They may take medications or narcotics. It's not a good situation.

3. Ozone cures pain — any pain.

Of all the things I've ever done in medicine, it is the most gratifying thing to take one of these patients who has been in chronic misery for so many years and within 15 minutes, they get up, start walking around the office, and tears start rolling down their face. They say something like, "Dr. Shallenberger, I've been suffering for 20 years with this. It's gone now. I can hardly remember not having this pain. Why the heck doesn't everybody do this?" I see these life-changing patient experiences so

often, especially with backs and necks that people have suffered with for so many years.

Last week, I had two people who came in to see me whom I had treated previously. In this case, it was their knees. They were told that they needed total knee replacements. They couldn't get around, play golf, or even go up and down stairs. Their lives were dramatically affected by this. We took the pain away in a heartbeat. They came back for their follow-up visit and were basically breaking down crying saying, "I've been suffering for years, and here's this simple therapy." That is the most gratifying thing I think any physician can do, to take a patient out of pain.

What's great about this therapy is if someone is having chronic pain in an area of his or her body, this not only takes away the pain. In most cases, it will literally heal the problem that is causing the pain. They won't need the total knee operation or another back surgery. You actually fixed the problem.

So many times, the reason the body won't heal is because it doesn't have adequate oxidation in the injured area. If the back won't heal and you have chronic back pain, it's because there's a lack of oxidation there. When we inject ozone into that area, we correct that and healing takes place. It's dramatic, wonderful, and almost miraculous. I have to say it's the most fun thing I can do.

DR. KONDROT: You are describing

injecting ozone directly into the painful area. Is that correct?

DR. SHALLENBERGER: Yes. It's exactly that. If the knee hurts, I inject into the knee. If they have a torn rotator cuff, I inject into the shoulder. If their neck hurts and they've had five surgeries, and they have metal in there, I will inject into the neck. If their ankle hurts, I inject into the ankle. It's pretty much as simple as that.

I would have to say it is rare when it doesn't really effectively help that person. That's why I think all doctors ought to know this.

DR. KONDROT: I know a lot of alternative doctors who use this technique, mainly because the number-one problem people have is that they're in pain. They go to their doctor because they want to get out of pain. Traditional medicine will put them on a narcotic or do surgery, which in many cases doesn't help.

I'm going to put you on the spot. Is this something that works on the majority of patients or on 50%?

DR. SHALLENBERGER: Let me put it to you this way. Normally I get patients when they've already had three surgeries and nothing is working. These are the kind of people I get. My patients are the ones who have bone-on-bone knee disease, and they've been told by their doctor that they need a total knee replacement. I don't get the easy ones.

I probably fix a good 85% of them. The rest of them will end up needing a total knee replacement or other surgery. I don't fix every single one of them because some of them are just way beyond repair by the time they get in. If every doctor out there knew this, and early on patients with bad knees would have this treatment, which takes a whole whopping three minutes and is entirely safe and inexpensive, I would venture to say there would be very few total knee replacements ever being done.

DR. KONDROT: I'm 63, and I'm still running marathons. Hopefully, I'm not going to need your services, but if I do start to get some knee problems, that would be the number-one treatment I'd receive. I want to avoid discomfort, aching, swelling, and difficulty walking. That makes sense to me.

DR. SHALLENBERGER: I had a guy come in last week. He told me, "I've had this chronic pain in my rotator cuff that's up in the shoulder. The doctor says he needs to replace my shoulder. I'm going to be out of work for three months. I can't do that. I've been suffering with this pain for two years because I can't take three months off for a shoulder surgery." We fixed him in three visits. He's out doing his thing and does not have a problem.

We also talk to patients about how they eat, what their stress is like, and the whole shebang about their lifestyle. We like to deal with all of that. But for their pain, we can just treat the area, and they'll see immediate results.

....

Frank Shallenberger, md, md(h), abaam

The Nevada Center of
Alternative & Anti-Aging Medicine
1231 Country Club Drive
Carson City, NV 89703
(775)884-3990
www.antiagingmedicine.com

Bruce H. Shelton, MD, MD(H), DiHom, FBIH

PHOENIX, ARIZONA

Interviewed July 14, 2013

1. This doctor was ready for disability because of his mold allergy until he found the cure, and now he shares it with others.

2. Having a root canal may save your tooth but kill you!

3. Why scars are way more than skin deep!

DR. KONDROT: It's a real pleasure to introduce Dr. Bruce Shelton. He has dedicated much of his life not only to homeopathy, but he's been the president of the Arizona Homeopathy Medical Association for the last nine years. He has helped lead the organization to assume prominence within the medical community in Arizona. I have succeeded him in this position and, my focus is on promoting homeopathy and alternative medicine throughout the United States and honoring those doctors who have contributed so much to homeopathy and integrative medicine. Dr. Shelton, it's great to have you on the *Top Alternative Doctors of America*.

DR. SHELTON: It's a definite pleasure to be here. I will tell you that in the two months since you've taken over, you've done such a good job. You've hit the ground running and have created this great show. I appreciate being here, and I congratulate you.

DR. KONDROT: Thank you. You and I both have something in common. We were introduced to homeopathy through our asthma. I wonder if you could share with us how you got interested in homeopathy, your career, the various organizations you belong to, positions you have held, and some background on your work.

DR. SHELTON: It's an involved story. First of all, I'm a graduate of New York Medical College. I moved to Arizona to do my internship and residency at Good Samaritan Hospital. For about 14 years, up to the late 1980s, I was a practicing board-certified MD family physician.

Then one day I woke up and I had a fever and a cough. I knew I was sick and went to the emergency room on the ground floor of our building. I had the doctor do a blood count and a chest X-ray, and it turned out that I had pneumonia. That scared me to death. Doctors aren't supposed to get sick. Pneumonia is serious.

The lung specialist said, "You probably have a simple community-acquired pneumonia." He put me on antibiotics and told me to go home and put my feet up for a week and relax, and everything would be okay.

I went back a week later and, sure enough, a repeat chest X-ray showed that the pneumonia was gone. But all of a sudden, I was wheezing. I developed asthma for the first time in my life. I took Theophylline, which is a drug for asthma. At the end of another week, I was much worse. I went back, and the doctor said, "I don't understand what's happening to you. Take this inhaler."

To make a long story short, a month went by and I was on six different drugs, including antihistamines, cortisone, and another round of antibiotics. Within a month, I became a pulmonary cripple. I was 40 years old at the time. That was 28 years ago. It was terrible. I couldn't think or work. The drugs were making my head sick. I went to another doctor to get a consult to see if there was anything else that could be done. He gave me another couple of drugs.

At the end of two to three months, I thought I was dying. I was in terrible shape. I couldn't work anymore, and I was getting ready to file my disability papers. It was a very scary experience for me because everything that could possibly be done was being done. I tell people that God sent me a magazine in the mail that was a medical journal. On the back cover was an ad for a medical conference to be held near Stanford University. It was sponsored by the Otolaryngic Allergy Academy, and the speaker was Dr. Vincent Marinkovich. Dr. Marinkovich specialized in diagnosing and treating mysterious ailments caused by household molds that baffled other doctors.

1. This doctor was ready for disability because of his mold allergy until he found the cure, and now he shares it with others.

I knew that was my answer, so I immediately made plans go to the conference. There I learned about a new way of testing for allergies using the Otolaryngic allergy method. It turned out that I was allergic to botrytis mold. Botrytis mold is the mold used to make wine sweeter. I was the head of a wine club. To help me recover, they made a dilute amount of this botrytis mold and put a couple of drops under my tongue. It was like a miracle. Within 20 minutes, my lungs opened up as if someone had pushed a button. I could breathe again. It was the epiphany of my life. It changed how I appreciated medicine. It sent me back to school to learn how to do what this doctor did with me. It changed my life.

I learned to practice Otolaryngic allergy, which literally is the allopathic model of homeopathy. It uses dilute amounts of the same things that make you sick, if you can figure out what that is. If you're allergic to tomatoes and you get headaches, a couple of drops of diluted tomatoes under your tongue will make the headaches go away.

It was a fascinating experience. I learned how to treat the flu by giving people diluted drops of flu vaccine, and their flu symptoms went away in a matter of hours. It was amazing.

I continued to take courses through the American Academy of Otolaryngic Allergy, which is the organization that ear, nose, and throat doctors have set up to treat allergy patients. I got to the end of the advanced course where I learned all types of techniques to treat food sensitivities, and I said, "There must be more to this. This is fascinating. I'm treating people I could never make better before."

I didn't understand what homeopathy was. I had heard the word before. It was almost like a dirty word in the medical profession, but I ended up learning homeopathy through Dr. Fuller Royal in Las Vegas. He's one of the leading homeopaths and one of the mentors of my life. I eventually enrolled in the British Institute of Homeopathy. Taking that course put me on the road to the rest of my career.

DR. KONDROT: Dr. Shelton, I wonder if you could tell us why your approach, called comprehensive homeopathy, is different from traditional homeopathy and why you use it exclusively in your practice.

DR. SHELTON: It's a very interesting topic. As I learned how to practice regular homeopathy, I focused on treating people's allergies. Then I learned about the work of Dr. Hans Heinrich Reckeweg through representatives of the company Heel. The most well-known medicine formulated by Dr. Reckeweg is Traumeel. If you talk about homeopathy, many people will say that they have used Traumeel. You can buy it over the counter in a health food store as a topical ointment for injuries and sprains. A lot of doctors inject it for people with arthritis and injury.

I went to all the meetings and became quite enamored with the use of combination remedies. Dr. Reckeweg combined multiple ingredients in a single product. Traumeel, as an example, has 12 different polychrest homeopathic remedies in its formula. A polychrest is a very strong-acting single remedy.

I really enjoyed these seminars, and I became one of Heel's bigger customers. As a result, I was invited to attend a conference in Baden-Baden, Germany, where I met people from all over the world including Dr. Garry Gordon, known for his pioneering work in chelation therapy and just about every type of integrative medicine.

We spent three days there, and I met several marketing people from Heel. They asked me to host a lecture for doctors here in Arizona. They liked what I did, and they hired me as one of their speakers. From about 1996 on, I must have gone to about 200 different seminars on behalf of Heel. I was eventually appointed their USA Chief Medical Director. It changed my life to get this second job. It was interesting, and I became the head of their speaker's bureau here in the United States. We would plan seminars and meetings about how homotoxicology could cure illnesses like asthma, urinary tract infections, prostate problems, gastrointestinal upsets, vision problem, mental problems, anxiety, arthritis, and fibromyalgia. Homotoxicology is a way of understanding illness as the body's failure to handle toxins and was introduced as a discipline by Dr. Reckeweg.

DR. KONDROT: I wonder if you could share with us what really impressed you about that meeting in Baden-Baden. What do you feel makes comprehensive homeopathy a better approach to treating disease than the more traditional homeopathy?

DR. SHELTON: Samuel Hahnemann, the father of classical homeopathy, said you can only use one remedy at a time. That is not the case. Dr. Reckeweg said if you have an eye problem, there may be ten different main remedies that are good for eye disease. In Dr. Hahnemann's world, you're supposed to choose one remedy and give that one remedy to the patient. What Dr. Reckeweg did was put all ten remedies into the same bottle, and the immune system of the patient selects the one it wants. It makes the practice of homeopathy much easier and therefore way more efficient.

The body has great innate intelligence, and the way Dr. Reckeweg designed the remedies is that certain remedies are good for certain things but have problems with other things. The patient may have eye watering and a headache. They may have eye watering and a stomachache. By combining a remedy that's good for your eyes but also good for your head or for your stomach, you get a multiple effect out of the treatment. You end up negating the side effects that might develop. The work of Dr. Reckeweg deserves a Nobel Prize.

I spent 15 years working with Heel which is a scientifically based company with laboratories, trained technicians, and sterile techniques. That impressed me. It was the real deal. The Heel Company is a subsidiary of the company that owns

BMW. It's a very wealthy company, and it spared no expense in doing things right. They did research and studies on many of their products. As far as homotoxicology went, when Dr. Reckeweg passed away in 1984, they stopped formulating new remedies. As things would have it, six or seven years ago, the American branch of Heel had a huge management shakeup, and things were not going well.

I was affiliated with another company called Deseret Biologicals in Utah. It's called DesBIO. I got very close with the CEO of DesBIO mainly because he was also involved with the electrodermal testing company, Biomeridian, that I worked with. He was the CEO of that company. He left it and bought Deseret Biologicals.

He offered me a job that would involve designing new remedies. The company was getting involved with a project called NAET, the Nambudripad Allergy Elimination Technique. Dr. Nambudripad is an acupuncturist and chiropractor who practices in Orange County, California. I was hired to help develop 28 new homeopathic combination remedies, which we ended up calling comprehensive homeopathy. Those remedies have been remarkable in how they help people. My work in the last six years has been remarkable in that I'm now able to help people with conditions that I wasn't able to help previously.

DR. KONDROT: We're going to be talking about another very interesting therapy that Dr. Shelton uses. It's called neural therapy. Dr. Shelton, please tell us what this is. You told me it has really changed the way you practice medicine.

DR. SHELTON: It was another one of those epiphanies along my career path. I told you that I was trained in homeopathy by Dr. Fuller Royal in Las Vegas. Dr. Royal is a great advocate of electrodermal testing. After he taught the homeopathic course and I bought my Interro device, which I used at the time to determine the correct homeopathic remedies, I said, "I can't go home until you test me."

2. Having a root canal may save your tooth but kill you!

He tested me, and he was looking at my results on his computer. He said, "Open your mouth." He looked inside my mouth and said, "You have a lot of fillings." At that time, I had 16 mercury amalgam fillings in my mouth from my childhood which no one ever did anything about. Dr. Royal had told me that if I didn't take my fillings out, I'd have a heart attack within a year or two based on the teeth that were affected by these fillings. That's all I had to hear.

I went to see Dr. Terry Lee in Phoenix. Dr. Lee looked at me. I was a medical doctor coming to him with dental issues, which is something he was very excited about. Most medical doctors don't believe that mercury is bad for you.

Soon I attended the American Academy of Biological Dentistry Conference and heard a lecturer named Dr. Dietrich Klinghardt. Dr. Klinghardt is a German medical doctor who is one of the leading advocates of neural therapy. Neural therapy started off with injections into scars. A scar of any kind disconnects the skin from the acupuncture meridian at the spot the scar transects the point. This needs to be reconnected. The thing that reconnects them is injecting the scar superficially with Novocain and vitamin B12. You have no idea the effect that it has. You can make migraine headaches go away practically instantaneously. You can treat aches and pains, asthma, gastrointestinal disease. You name the illness. If you inject the correct points with the neural therapy formulas of vitamin B12 and procaine, you can resolve a lot of issues.

3. Why scars are way more than skin deep!

I ask each patient who comes into my office if they have scars. The original scar the patient has is their belly button. Nowadays, we've learned how to treat scars with lasers. We have a laser in our office for people who don't want to be injected with a needle. It does similar things.

The use of neural therapy to treat the acupuncture points that are involved offers a whole atlas of points you can treat for different types of illnesses. There are different ganglion areas of the autonomic nervous system that you can inject. You can inject homeopathic remedies into these points. You can literally resolve issues on the spot that patients have had for years.

Maybe a patient has had a sore shoulder for a long time, and they also have a scar on their arm from a cut they got ten years earlier. They don't see the connection. You inject that scar on their arm with a little bit of infiltrated procaine and B12, and all of a sudden they can raise their arm above shoulder level, when they couldn't have done it before. They've been to chiropractors, acupuncturists, physical therapists, and all of a sudden you've fixed their scars and they get better.

I know you've used neural therapy by injecting into people's eye sockets. Dr. Klinghardt did it to me once. He actually went into the little point under my eye. It was like someone had sewn the Mount Palomar telescope onto my face the way my vision changed. The colors were brighter. My vision cleared.

I know you've done things like injecting ozone. Some of the things you've done that I've watched are amazing because you're into eye treatment.

That's neural therapy. It all comes from Austria where it was discovered by a Dr. Huneke many years ago.

DR. KONDROT: I want to back up a little bit because you began to speak about having your dental amalgams addressed. I understand that a good part of your practice, even though you're not a dentist, is focused on the teeth. I wonder if you could talk a little bit about your understanding in terms of pathology and looking at the teeth amalgams, root canals, etc.

DR. SHELTON: Every tooth in your mouth sits on a different acupuncture meridian. We have a chart in our office that shows the different organ connections of every tooth. People who have had root canals usually have infections underneath the tooth socket. Depending on which tooth that is, that's the organ where they usually have their illness.

I have a lot of people come in who tell me they have ulcerative colitis or breast disease. I say, "Let me look in your mouth." Sure enough, there's a cap on the fifth tooth to the right or left of the midline. When I ask them what is under the cap, they say it's a root canal, needed because of an infection. After they tell me their health problem, I usually tell them that it is in a part of their body connected to the tooth with the root canal.

In our office, we use thermography to measure the heat that comes off the skin overlying areas of inflammation. We take a picture of the person's head. If we see hot spots in their jaw, I look in their mouth and know they have a dental foci, like they've had a wisdom tooth pulled that didn't have the socket cleaned out properly, or a root canal, which is the worst thing they can have, or a horribly corroded mercury filling that turns black and doesn't look silvery anymore; that calls for an immediate referral to someone in the biological dental world.

You have no idea how many patients have been to top allopathic doctors, including major clinics in Arizona, who have spent $20,000 or $30,000 trying to find answers to horrible illness. The clinic ends up giving up, and they send the patients home with Prozac and cortisone. They say, "Go have a good life. We can't help you."

They come into my office, and I tell them about homeopathy. Then we do a thermogram. If we see a hot spot in their mouth, we refer them to a dentist. There they have dental imaging procedures, usually done with ultrasound and a device called a Cavitat. I've seen patients get better in the dental chair. Then they come back in, and we clean them up with our detox procedures using our comprehensive homeopathic remedies, of which we have several hundred.

Combining what I do with biological dentistry has literally allowed me to treat illnesses that a regular doctor doesn't have any answers for. They just give people antidepressants, tranquilizers, and pain medicine.

My patients get homeopathic care and answers. It's one of the few specialties in medicine where, if you come up with the right remedy — which is no guarantee — you can cure people.

In medicine, the word "cure" is a big no-no. I've seen cures be effected by simple things like dilute amounts of substances that would make the patient sick in large amounts, which is the basis of homeopathy in the first place. We've treated people's scars, teeth, and points in their acupuncture meridians which are connected to the different organs. We get great results. I know you've seen it too in your own practice.

DR. KONDROT: That's the beauty of homeopathy. In homeopathy, we look at the underlying cause of disease. In your case, you had a severe case of pneumonia that led to asthma. No one looked at the underlying cause, which turned out to be that particular mold. I wonder if you could comment on sanum therapy, which is another big part of your practice.

DR. SHELTON: It is. A lot of my epiphanies have come from listening to major teachers. There are amazing doctors around the world who know things that are not in the mainstream. I envied them after I listened to them because I'd never heard of these techniques before.

Another great lecturer who has changed my life as a physician is Dr. Thomas Rau, MD of Switzerland. Dr. Rau is the world expert on teaching sanum therapies, the work of Dr. Gunther Enderlein.

We all know that if you take antibiotics or some other drugs, the supposedly good germs that live in our intestines get neutralized somehow, and you need to take acidophilus in order to replace them so your body can work.

I always ask, "Do you ever wonder why bugs live inside of us?" The answer is that when we were created, we were not given all the enzymes we need to totally digest our food. In its place, this friendly little species of fungus in its baby form was allowed to live inside of us. These little baby bugs have the enzymes that

help digest the food. The problem is that when the terrain of our body — terrain being defined as acid-base balance, mineral balance and oxygen balance — goes out of balance, the little bugs change their forms or morph and become bigger, badder bugs. They become viral forms, bacterial forms, and major fungal forms.

By the time we're growing these little germs inside of us, the body's immune system kicks in and tries to neutralize them. They are the debris from that fight that causes all of our chronic degenerative diseases like hardening of the arteries, arthritis, fibromyalgia, and cancer.

The answer to solving the problem is fixing the terrain. You have to get the heavy metals out through chelation. That is a whole major focus of my practice. You need to fix the acid-base balance, and you need to put the right nutrition back in the body so the oxygen balance becomes normal.

The other way to deal with it is through a line of homeopathic products called the sanum remedies that were developed by Dr. Enderlein. They are homeopathic dilutions of the little germ forms that the good bugs morph into. When you fix the terrain and take these homeopathic sanum remedies, the bugs un-morph, and the body can heal.

The best doctor a patient is ever going to have is their own immune system. Getting it back to normal is the best way to go. That is what sanum therapy is all about. It's neutralizing the bad bugs back to their baby forms because there's no way to kill them.

Antibiotics do not do anything except morph bacteria into fungus and make you sick. What you need to do is get the bacteria, virus, and fungus back to their preforms. Once you do that, then you will focus on good nutrition. You're not going to mess your terrain up any longer. You're going to stay healthy for the rest of your life by doing this. That's the goal of comprehensive therapy: putting all these pieces of the puzzle together, which is something we do.

DR. KONDROT: You have one of the most fascinating practices that I have come across with the various therapies you use. The bottom line is the results you're getting. You're really helping a lot of people.

DR. KONDROT: Let's close by talking about another interesting aspect of your practice, red wine.

DR. SHELTON: As I told you in the beginning, I got sick from the botrytis mold which was blowing out of my wine room into my bedroom. I became very fascinated as the commander of the Arizona chapter of the Brotherhood of the Knights of the Vine in using wine for medical uses.

Many doctors in history have cured people by having them drink wine. I actually had a goal at one point in time to help people diet and lose weight by writing a book called *The Dr. Shelton*

Wine Diet. I've never been able to put it together in its absolute final form because it takes a great amount of research and willpower in order to not get hungry when you drink wine.

Wine is the most healthful and hygienic of beverages. It's mentioned over 450 times in the Bible *and* it does prevent heart disease. For people who don't drink, there are things like resveratrol, which is a supplement made from the skin of wine grapes, which are very high in the phenolics that are helpful as antioxidants to prevent abnormal blood clotting. A glass of wine a day keeps the heart doctor away. It's been my great interest to someday write about it and attract people to that interest in my life.

DR. KONDROT: With the last couple of minutes remaining, do you have any closing comments for the listeners?

DR. SHELTON: I've decided to add injectable hormone pellet therapy to my practice as a modern form of hormone replacement therapy or HRT. Each pellet that is placed under the skin slowly releases hormones into the system as our homeopathic methods are rejuvenating stressed adrenal glands. The pellets last four to five months before remeasurements are needed to determine a next dose. It's proven to be a safe technique that sure beats twice daily hormone pill replacement and/or messy creams that can rub off onto the skin of your partner and masculinize or feminize the partner as the case might be.

I consider medicine and health workups as a six-part puzzle. I tell people that the main constitutional single homeopathic remedy is like the ignition key that goes in your car which is puzzle piece number one. If it's the right key and it's really your car, it should start the motor. If, however, you are missing sparkplugs in the engine, the car won't start. This equates to missing nutrition and is puzzle piece number two. If you've got sand in your oil line, which is heavy metal toxicity (puzzle piece three), the car won't start either. If you've got dental problems (puzzle piece four), which is the teeth connection *and* if you've got abnormal germs in your system, which is the sanum connection (puzzle piece five), or if your muscles and bones are out of place (puzzle piece six), that's where you need neuromuscular integration which is chiropractic/osteopathic and/or neural therapy.

A chiropractor who works with me in my office ends up seeing a lot of my patients. I refer to osteopaths and chiropractors because it's a six-part puzzle and all six pieces need to be covered in order to treat the patients appropriately. With that said, along with proper nutrition, as you noted in your *10 Essentials to Save your Sight* book, the patient gets all their puzzle pieces covered. I think your book is necessary reading for many patients. It talks about eye disease, but nutrition and living right and doing all the right healthy things you discuss are very important to your health.

....

BRUCE H. SHELTON, MD, MD(H), DIHOM, FBIH

VALLEY INTEGRATIVE PHYSICIANS PLLC

14231 N 7th Street

Phoenix, AZ 85022

(602)504-1000 fax (602)504-1008

www.drbruceshelton.com

shelton@drbruceshelton.com

Mark Starr, MD, MD(H)

PARADISE VALLEY, ARIZONA

Interviewed October 8, 2013

1. **When they switched patients from the synthetic to the glandular thyroid, their symptoms greatly improved.**

2. **All you have to do is breathe, eat, and drink water these days, and you become poisoned.**

3. **None of my patients on a full dose of thyroid, which is over 2 grains, has ever had a heart attack.**

DR. KONDROT: Dr. Mark Starr is the author of two books. One, which is a favorite of mine, is *Hypothyroidism Type 2: The Epidemic*. This book is on my shelf, and any time I see patients whom I suspect have some type of thyroid problem, I tell them, "You've got to read Mark Starr's book." Now he's coming out with another book. Will you share with us a little bit about your background and how you got interested in alternative medicine? Most of us who have been doing alternative medicine started out like traditional doctors, and we thought we had all the answers.

DR. STARR: Yes, and so did I. I had chronic back pain from high school due to a fractured low back. I was a running back, and I was tackled. I started to get up, and a guy hit me with his shoulder pads right in my low back and fractured it. They offered surgery in 1968 or '69, but luckily for me, the orthopedist said, "Mark, the surgeries don't work so well, so you might as well do some exercises." A laminectomy was the procedure they performed back then. I went into Physical Medicine and Rehabilitation after medical school because of my chronic back pain. Physical Medicine and Rehabilitation includes conservative treatment for back and neck pain.

I was ten years behind everybody else in medical school. I had always wanted to be a doctor, but I had a bad motorcycle accident when I was 20. I didn't finish med school until I was 37 and, by the time I was finishing residency, at the age of 40, I was getting chilly easily, my concentration was declining, and I had joint and muscle pain, and not just in my back. My skin was dry, and I had a number of symptoms associated with low thyroid. Of course, I knew about hypothyroidism, and my older brother and mother were already taking synthetic thyroid. I sought help from my colleagues at the University of Missouri, but they would not treat me because my thyroid blood tests were normal. I certainly didn't know how to treat myself back then.

Fortunately for me, I heard a medical doctor lecture at our national conference about trigger-point injections and muscle pain. I went to study with him. He was chairman of the Bronx Veteran's Hospital rehab department. I had planned on staying six weeks after completing my residency, and I ended up staying two years. One of the reasons was because, after spending a year at the Bronx Veteran's Hospital, I went over to learn from *his* teacher.

My teacher was 66 at the time, and

his teacher was 90 and still working two days a week. His name was Hans Kraus. He treated President Kennedy's low-back pain and got rid of it after Kennedy had already had three failed back surgeries. He treated Jonas Salk, Yul Brynner, and Katharine Hepburn. At age 90, he was attracting a lot of people from the United Nations, and he had a worldwide following.

When I went to see him, I still had some back pain despite lots of trigger-point injections for a year. I told him my story and he said, "You need to go see Dr. Sonkin." Larry Sonkin was an MD, PhD at the New York Hospital Cornell Endocrinology Clinic where they invented the Pap smear, and they thought they were the number-one hormone place on the planet. During my first visit, Dr. Sonkin examined me and heard my story and said, "You need thyroid." I said, "How can that be since my blood tests have been normal?" He said, "Mark, I hate to tell you, but the blood tests are missing millions of patients who are low thyroid, and you're one of them." I'll be darned if he didn't put me on thyroid and, within a short period of time, most of my symptoms started resolving.

After two years in New York, I started a pain clinic in Columbia, Missouri, where I had gone to med school and lived for 20 years. Within two years, I realized that most of my pain patients had the same thing I did, which was low thyroid. I started trying to prove this fact because I rapidly became a pariah for treating my patients who had normal thyroid studies, and the insurance companies wouldn't pay for what I did. I no longer take insurance because I lost over $100,000 after five years in my first practice.

Insurance companies said that my treatment was not standard of care, and they even turned down my muscle-pain injections because I didn't use any steroids. Then Medicare would pay about $10 for the physical therapy my patients required. I decided that I was never going to make a living doing what I wanted if something didn't change. What I learned in New York and practiced in my pain clinic offered cures that I never imagined to be possible. So, I wrote a book that required five and a half years of research. A lot of that research is on my website, www.21CenturyMed.com, and you can see before and after treatment pictures. You can change the way people look quite profoundly when they are treated for hypothyroidism.

The last medical textbook I could find that had before and after treatment pictures was published 1957. The doctor was president of The American Endocrine Society. One of his case studies was the resolution of congestive heart failure with thyroid. I found out about Dr. Broda Barnes' work and his research foundation in 1998. He was an MD, PhD Endocrinologist who earned his PhD in 1930 and then became a medical doctor in 1937. He did more research than anybody on our planet for the next 50 years. He died in the 1980s in his 80s. The web site for

his research foundation is www.Broda-Barnes.org.

One of his books was called *Solved: The Riddle of Heart Attacks*. It came out in 1975. He reviewed 70,000 consecutive autopsy reports in Graz, Austria, where Marie Antoinette's mother, Queen Maria Theresa, mandated everybody have autopsies from the late 1700s because the state of health was so poor there. There was a treasure trove of information, and he spent 18 summers going through 70,000 autopsies.

Here was all the evidence about how to prevent heart attacks. He did a 20-year study that included over 1,500 patients. His patients should have had 74 heart attacks based on the average number in America. Only four people had a heart attack. That was over a 90% reduction in heart attacks in a 20-year study, yet none of his research is taught in medical school or in any formal medical training. You don't get reimbursed if you follow his protocol, so it's a big problem.

DR. KONDROT: Could you go into a little more detail about the symptoms of hypo-thyroidism? It's kind of shocking to me that the lab studies really don't mean anything, so a physician has to depend more on the symptoms. Many doctors, as you bring out in your book, don't pay attention to the symptoms and just rule out hypothyroid based on the lab tests.

DR. STARR: For 40 years now, doctors have been treating lab tests instead of patients, and have they ever missed the boat with that. The thyroid controls our body's metabolism, the speed and efficiency at which each and every one of our cells work. When you're low thyroid or hypothyroid, the metabolism slows down. Some of the more common symptoms are fatigue and weakness, cold intolerance, joint and muscle pain, depression, muscle cramps, headaches, menstrual problems, infertility, dental problems, and ADHD in children. These children don't need Ritalin to speed them up; they need thyroid treatment to speed them up.

Problems during pregnancy are also often due to low thyroid, excess weight gain and pre-eclampsia. Alzheimer's and dementia may be due to hypothyroidism. You have an increased risk of cancer if you have hypothyroidism.

There have been four generations of endocrinologists in one Belgian family, the Hertoghe family. The Belgium doctors did a study in which they switched patients from the synthetic thyroid which they found not nearly as effective to the old fashioned pig thyroid which is what they used the first half of the 20th century, and quite successfully.

1. When they switched patients from the synthetic to the glandular thyroid, their symptoms greatly improved.

They had a number of patients who came to their clinic who were complaining of low thyroid despite being treated by other doctors who had placed them on Levothyroxine, Levoxyl, or Synthroid.

These are all T4, one form of thyroid hormone. Doctors have been taught to use T4 for 40 years.

They switched them from their synthetic drug to the old-fashioned pig thyroid, or glandular type of thyroid, which is how the first cure was found out in 1891. By the early 1900s, they had before and after treatment pictures and a whole host of research way back when.

When they switched patients from the synthetic, fatigue was reduced by 90% of the patients who came in on the synthetic stuff to 26% after two years. The cold intolerance went from 86% to 23%. Joint and muscle pain went from 77% to 28%, so you can get rid of two thirds of joint and muscle pain. Headaches went from 55% to 15%. That includes migraines, so a vast majority of joint and muscle pain and migraines will resolve just by using thyroid properly. After I stopped taking insurance, the patients couldn't afford my fancy injections and physical therapy any more. Using enough glandular thyroid reversed two thirds of my patients' joint and muscle pain. Most of the migraines and headaches also resolved.

DR. KONDROT: The question I have is why is the pig thyroid is so much better than the synthetic? What's the explanation for that?

DR. STARR: Actually sheep, beef, and pigs' thyroid worked way back when. They're using different forms of glandular thyroid. It's called Armour, or at least it used to be.

There are different forms of Armour these days. It was the Armour Meat Company that produced the pig thyroid.

There are four different types of thyroid hormones. The one that everybody is given, which is the most abundantly produced by our own thyroid, is called T4. The pig thyroid has T4 but it also has T3, which is five times as potent as the T4. Basically, the main activity of the thyroid in the whole body is done by T3 which doctors have been taught not to use now for over 40 years. The pig thyroid also has T2, which is shown to have some efficacy, and T1, so it has all four types of thyroid hormone.

I learned that anybody with Hashimoto's, which is an autoimmune thyroid problem when the body is attacking its own thyroid and is becoming quite epidemic, you have to use the synthetics. Adding more pig thyroid, which is identical to our own thyroid, just makes the problem worse because your body is already attacking your own thyroid gland when you have Hashimoto's. I have a chapter on that in my already-published book.

DR. KONDROT: You recommend the Armour over the synthetic.

DR. STARR: I recommend Armour, Nature-Throid, or Westhroid. There used to be generic desiccated thyroid but the FDA seemed to make it harder and harder to come by. That's what I'm on — the pig thyroid — and have been for 15 years.

DR. KONDROT: You gave a lot of symptoms, and I would say that probably 80% to 90% of the population has one or more of those symptoms.

DR. STARR: Broda Barnes, who died in the 1980s in his 80s, published a book that's still available because people want to know why they're sick. It's called *Hypothyroidism: The Unsuspected Illness.* In that book he said, at the time that it was published in 1976, that 40% of Americans had low thyroid, and in ten more years it would be 50%, because half the population that was hypothyroid formerly died of infections before they became symptomatic.

Autopsies showed that as the rate of infections declined; of course, the symptoms associated with low thyroid became pervasive because for thousands of years, more than two thirds of the population would get picked off at a relatively young age from plague, smallpox, and tuberculosis. Only when we introduced antibiotics and anti-tubercular drugs in 1945 did the hypothyroid population grow, and the condition become epidemic.

DR. KONDROT: Can you talk a little bit about other contributory factors, such as environmental factors that are essentially destroying our hormonal system and, in particular, the thyroid? In my ophthalmology practice, I think that hypothyroidism is linked to conditions like glaucoma and macular degeneration, so this is a very serious problem that should be investigated if you're having health issues.

DR. STARR: My book has an environmental chapter that I worked on for a whole year. I had a lot of first-hand experience with that, too. My mother was unfortunately highly allergic to the marlex mesh and prolene sutures that were placed inside of her pelvis for reconstructive surgery for rectal and bladder prolapse. The prolene and marlex are basically plastic. Nobody in Missouri could figure out what was wrong with her. Luckily she made it to the Environmental Health Center, but she was nearly dead by the time she got there.

The Environmental Health Center in Dallas is the number-one place for environmental medicine in the whole world. Dr. Rea is a cardiothoracic surgeon who became chemically sensitive and has treated about 50,000 patients. I learned quite a bit about environmental medicine, and he and Theo Colborn, who authored *Our Stolen Future*, helped guide me in my research.

There is a really good study that has been done twice now by the environmental working group, www.ewg.org. They tested the umbilical cord blood of women all over the country for toxins. It's a very sophisticated test with disturbing results. Babies are being bathed in over 200 nasty neurotoxins, carcinogens, and birth-defect-causing chemicals before they're born.

DR. KONDROT: You wonder what chance a newborn baby has being exposed to all of those toxins.

2. All you have to do is breathe, eat, and drink water these days, and you become poisoned.

DR. STARR: I have to tell you that the children are getting sicker and sicker progressively, in my opinion. That's what I've seen for 15 years now and it's not good. I do the best I can to enlighten everybody because what we do to the planet, we do to ourselves. The toxins are ubiquitous. They go from the North Pole to the South Pole and every place in between, so all you have to do is breathe, eat, and drink water these days, and you become poisoned. Now we have Fukushima where the radioactive iodine and radioactive cesium continue to spew into the Pacific Ocean. For instance, they found a large tuna that had apparently migrated from Fukushima within six or twelve months of the disaster, and it had a lot of radioactive cesium, which produces gamma rays and is extraordinarily dangerous. What did the FDA do about the fact that the tuna had radioactive cesium? They raised the safe levels to the highest in the world so they could keep selling their radioactive cesium-infested tuna fish. I tell my patients not to eat Pacific seafood anymore. That's a shame, and some of the Alaskan fish have also been contaminated.

The Chernobyl research showed that

the radioactive cesium goes right for the hormone-producing tissues in the heart. It is in the food chain over in Russia, and only 20% of the children around Chernobyl are healthy. Many are dying of heart failure and have all sorts of birth defects and problems.

My brother is an antinuclear specialist and he has an article called *Costs and Consequences of the Fukushima Daiichi Disaster*. You can find that if you do a Google search. His name is Steven Starr. He has presented lectures at the General Assembly of the United Nations and has contacts all over the world. He keeps me apprised of the latest radiation news, which isn't good.

Plastic bottles leech something called phthalates. Even the pediatricians are worried about it. You're not supposed to use plastic bottles because they leech the phthalates, which block thyroid hormone and don't do so well for other hormones either.

DR. KONDROT: A lot of parents microwave the plastic bottle and give it to their babies.

DR. STARR: I know. That's extremely toxic stuff. The good news is if you stop drinking out of plastic bottles, the phthalates are gone within several days. The bad news is that a whole lot of folks drink it every day. One thing you can do is stay informed with the wonderful website www.OurStolenFuture.com. There are pesticides, herbicides, fungi-

cides, flame-retardants, mercury, lead, arsenic, and all sorts of things that block thyroid function. Unfortunately, unless a person has been rigorously detoxified, everybody is toxic these days.

DR. KONDROT: Do you have some favorite methods of detoxification or perhaps some suggestions for the worst of those? Are there some supplements people can take to help decrease their toxic load?

DR. STARR: Dr. Rea at the Environmental Health Center in Dallas has been helping patients detoxify for decades now, and his main treatment is sauna. Only porcelain saunas are used at his clinic, due to possible cedar allergies, and they use a number of supplements. The one I recommend the most is something called The Gift from Mother Earth at www.MotherEarthLabs.com. The Gift and fulvic acid are two of the healthiest things on the planet. Fulvic acid is the most complicated molecule ever found in nature. There are about 50 pages in research studies on it on the website for Mother Earth Labs. It's potent stuff, but that's my favorite treatment. The Gift has humic and fulvic acid. People take that either before or right after the saunas because you're going to lose good minerals. If you don't sweat much, which is another sign of low thyroid as well as a sign of being toxic, you have to go very gradually and be very careful.

DR. KONDROT: Probably the most

important thing is to really look at your diet.

DR. STARR: Yes. I try to eat as much organic as I can. I have studies in my book, *Hypothyroidism Type 2,* on how chemicals in the foods that are not organic get into your blood stream, and yes, they do affect you. The mainstream literature says, "There's no difference," but yes, we do have studies showing there's a big difference. *Our Stolen Future* has a lot of good ways to try to avoid all of the pitfalls of our modern planet. The fulvic acid even reverses a lot of the radiation toxicity. It really is remarkable stuff.

DR. KONDROT: I know you're really excited about your latest book. Has that been released?

3. None of my patients on a full dose of thyroid, which is over 2 grains, has ever had a heart attack.

DR. STARR: It's going to be my first e-book. It's called *How to Prevent Heart Attacks.* None of my patients on a full dose of thyroid, which is over 2 grains, has ever had a heart attack. Most people don't realize that almost all the complications of diabetes are due to hardening of the arteries. When you give back the thyroid hormone, it stops. The diabetics have accelerated hardening of the arteries just like hypothyroid patients do. Dr. Barnes did a lot of research on that and thinks that diabetes may in large part be

due to hypothyroidism. For instance, I've only had three patients develop diabetes in my 15 years of prescribing thyroid, and all three were not yet on a full dose of thyroid.

Over 8% of Americans have the illness now, so not only can you stop the progression of hardening of the arteries, which causes all of the gangrene, amputations, blindness, kidney failure, and heart attacks, you can stop the complications of diabetes. I will have a YouTube video with a testimonial from a Type 1 diabetic woman. I guess I shouldn't say how old she is, but she went from being extremely fatigued and feeling quite poorly to riding up to 70 miles in a bicycle race that very year. She works out for two hours every day, so she has her life back.

DR. KONDROT: Mark, let's continue our discussion on hypothyroid disease. Let's talk a little bit about some of the methods you use to diagnose whether someone does indeed have a hypothyroid problem.

DR. STARR: Before I ever heard about Broda Barnes and his research foundation, my teacher, Larry Sonkin, MD, was in his 70s when he was treating me and teaching me. He showed me his research, which involved doing basal metabolic tests, which is how they diagnosed patients for decades before they came up with a blood test. Basal metabolism is what the thyroid controls. The patient would fast from about 8:00 at night until the morning when they would get up, and they would stick a tube in the patient's mouth, put a nose clip on him, and measure how much oxygen he inspired and CO_2 he expired, Then they could tell whether your metabolism was normal for your age, height, weight, and sex.

If your metabolism was low, plus if you had the symptoms of hypothyroidism, then you would get treatment. Dr. Barnes realized that the basal metabolism test was only about 75% accurate, so it wouldn't pick up everybody. A lot of people are tense or have pain and they wouldn't be able to relax; their temperature would be higher or their metabolism would be normal or even above normal, and yet they still needed thyroid, so he started testing the basal temperature. He did 1,000 Army recruits in World War II, and he tested a lot of the medical students that he was teaching at the University of Colorado. He published a paper in the *Journal of the American Medical Association* around 1942 called "Basal Temperature Versus Basal Metabolism" and showed that the basal temperature test was over 90% accurate.

All of the old endocrinologists knew that one of the many cardinal signs of low thyroid was low temperature. You put a thermometer under your arm in the morning and it should be at least 97.8 degrees. Women have to do it during their menstrual cycle. Days two, three, and four are the most accurate. Children and older women can do it any time and so can men. If you have an infection, of course, that will elevate your tempera-

ture, and that's not a good time to do it.

It's not 100% accurate. I saw one 30-year-old who had had emphysema for five years and was disabled both mentally and physically. She was thoroughly myxedematous, which is the medical term for hypothyroidism, and she recovered a whole lot of her health when I put her on thyroid, but her temperature was always elevated.

DR. KONDROT: This is something average people can do on their own. They just can buy a thermometer and check their temperature in the morning.

DR. STARR: That's right. Unfortunately, in all of the medical textbooks, the doctors have been taught that the basal temperature is not accurate. They have no references for this opinion; they just make that statement.

Myxedema is the medical term. Myx is for mucin. Mucin is the Greek word. Mucin is the normal constituent of our connective tissue, and in over half the patients with hypothyroidism, it accumulates in abnormal amounts. The edema is a firm type of swelling, so the medical term for hypothyroidism is called myxedema.

You can see the myxedema in these patients before treatment, and then after the treatment, their countenance or their whole appearance has changed completely. As I said, the last textbook that I could find that had before and after treatment pictures was in 1957.

Dr. Lisser was President of the American Endocrine Society. I will be featuring some of his work in my upcoming book as well. In Dr. Barnes' study on heart attacks where he decreased heart attacks over 90%, the dosages of the desiccated thyroid ranged from 2 grains to 5 grains.

In the Hertoghe study, a lot of the symptoms resolved by switching from the synthetic thyroid to the old-fashioned desiccated thyroid. The third-generation Belgian endocrinologist, Dr. Hertoghe, did a study on a couple hundred patients, and the average dose was 3 to 3.5 grains for adults. Similarly, it ranged from 2 grains to 5 grains just like Broda Barnes' study did. Not only that, the Hertoghes actually have a wonderful way to diagnose hypothyroidism on a 24-hour urine T3 test.

We have those tests in America, but the people who designed them tested patients whom they considered normal because they had normal thyroid tests and seemed to be relatively healthy. But the incidence of low thyroid is so pervasive that I don't think their test results are accurate because they took too many people who had low thyroid as a part of their normal study.

Unfortunately, we really don't have a good scientific test, and yet there is a lot of money being made by testing for thyroid problems. Not only that, but it's hard to convince endocrinologists who have been treating based on the same blood tests for 40 years that what they have been taught was wrong. They have a lot of certificates on their walls and have been treating for decades. This is a global problem. I have a friend in Canada who has been sanctioned for using desiccated thyroid. I have a friend in Sweden who told me that doctors there are duty bound to treat with synthetic thyroid for a year. If the patients still have a problem, they can make a special application to treat with the old-fashioned desiccated thyroid, yet they still are bound to use the TSH first.

When you use the TSH, the maximum dosage is only 1.5 to 2 grains, and 2 grains was the minimum dosage required in both Dr. Barnes' and the Hertoghe study. In my patients for the last 15 years, just like the Hertoghe study, the average dose for adults has been 3 to 3.5 grains.

Of course Dr. Barnes said, "The bigger the beast, the bigger the bullet." I have treated some 300-pound patients and they needed 5 or even 6 grains. Armour Thyroid used to make 5-grain tablets. I've been very fortunate to be able to have a homeopathic license, so my colleagues actually refer patients to me instead of sending me nasty notes and emails like I received during my first ten years in practice. I'm very grateful to have an MD(H) license. My website has a lot of information about this subject, and my book is also available there.

Dr. Mark Starr, MD, MD(H)
10565 N. Tatum Blvd B-115
Paradise Valley AZ 85253
(480)607-6503
www.21centurymed.com
mstarrmd@21centurymed.com

David Steenblock, DO

MISSION VIEJO, CA

Interviewed August 18, 2013

1. **I have developed a wide range of different techniques for treating people with difficult-to-treat problems.**

2. **If we give healthy, fresh stem cells to a person with cerebral palsy, the patient and family will most likely see improvements.**

3. **The best results with stem cells are achieved when they are given within the first ten days after a stroke.**

DR. KONDROT: Dr. David Steenblock is one of the leading world authorities on stem cell therapy of all types having treated over 5,000 patients with bone marrow transplants, fat stem cells, or umbilical cord stem cells. Dr. Steenblock was trained as a biochemist, a pathologist, a surgeon, a physician, and research scientist and has taken care of over 50,000 patients over the past 43 years. For the last ten years, he has specialized in the use of stem cells to treat a great variety of medical and health problems that otherwise were untreatable and incurable. Stem cells are a very hot topic for anyone who has any kind of chronic health problem since the results have been phenomenal for a great variety of different difficult to treat medical problems.

Dr. Steenblock is also the author of the first book for the public on the clinical use of umbilical cord-derived stem cell therapies. I recommend this book to anyone who wants a good understanding of stem cells. It's called *Umbilical Cord Stem Cell Therapy*, and it can be ordered by calling 1-800-300-1063.

He's also the creator of a stem cell enhancing product called Stemgevity, which increases the number of stem cells in your blood stream while also increasing the stem cell's strength. We have a lot of exciting things to talk about. Let's begin by your telling us a little bit about your medical career and how you got interested in alternative and integrative treatments.

DR. STEENBLOCK: It started many years ago with my own health problems. From the beginning of my life, I suffered from chronic allergies, low blood sugar, and chronic fatigue. I sought the help of different doctors through the years, but I didn't feel much improvement. Finally, I went to the very best allergy doctors at Case Western Reserve and spent quite a bit of time, energy, and a lot of pain at their hands trying to get some relief from my symptoms. After many months of suffering from weekly allergy shots, it became obvious that the conventional medical establishment did not have answers for me. I started to think of where else I could get help.

The first place I thought of was health food stores. I decided to go and visit one to see for myself what they were all about. I was amazed to find such a plethora of different substances that I had never heard of being used for treatments. That really intrigued me. I started studying all the nutritional and herbal books and articles that I could find. I started to apply things

that I read, started to change my diet, started adding supplements, started to exercise, and changed my environment. Within six months, I went from a health cripple to having vibrant health. I've been healthy ever since!

DR. KONDROT: It's kind of interesting, Dr. Steenblock. So many alternative doctors develop an interest in alternative treatments because of their own personal health issues. It seems like in many respects traditional medicine has let us down. Because of that, we then develop a passion for truly helping people who maybe are not getting the right answers from conventional medical circles. Let's talk a little bit more about how your practice then evolved into the alternative treatments that you're currently doing.

DR. STEENBLOCK: I was trained as a biochemist and pathologist as well as a physician. I did a rotating internship, which gave me a broad scope of experience that included general medical practice, internal medicine, emergency room medicine, surgery, ob-gyn, and orthopedics. Then, I became a sole practitioner in a rural logging town in Washington where I was in charge of a 32-bed hospital. Then, I went back into residency and studied four years in anatomical and clinical pathology so I could better understand the basic mechanisms of disease. This type of deep insight in the mechanisms of how diseases develop and injure the body gave me the understanding I needed to treat patients based on fixing the cause(s) of the conditions the person was suffering from rather than just prescribing another drug.

DR. KONDROT: What makes your practice special? What do you do differently? There are many really good alternative doctors out there, but everybody has a different approach. What is yours?

1. I have developed a wide range of different techniques for treating people with difficult-to-treat problems.

DR. STEENBLOCK: First, it's education. I have six more years of academic training than the average doctor. Second, I have a broad overview of medicine because I did the rotating internship, four years of pathology, and the surgical training. Third, I spent 40 years doing alternative medicine, often dealing with patients who could not be helped by other doctors. That's 40,000 or 50,000 patients, who virtually couldn't be helped by anybody else. I saw a lot of different pathologies and developed different solutions for dealing with a wide spectrum of difficult-to-treat patients.

I have developed a wide range of different techniques for treating people with difficult-to-treat problems. We use hyperbaric oxygen, external counter pulsation (ECP), pulsed electromagnetic field therapy, chelation therapy, periodic acceleration, intravenous therapies, hyperthermia, intermittent hypoxia, bone marrow, fat, and other stem cell treatments, platelet-rich plasma treatments, and nutritional therapies.

We've gone from hyperbaric oxygen in the late 1980s for patients with stroke and traumatic injury to the use of stem cells. We've developed some new techniques on this procedure, and we're getting great results. I have many testimonials on www.youtube.com (type in "Dr. Steenblock") and www.stemcellmd.org.

Our clinic is geared around stem cells. Anything and everything we do is to promote stem cell growth, stem cell growth factors, and enhancing the circulation and engraftment of these growth factors and stem cells to repair and regenerate the different tissues that are damaged in the patient's body.

Besides hyperbaric and stem cells, we have therapies like external counter-pulsation, which enhances the collateral circulation of the body, reduces hardening of the arteries, and increases oxygen to the heart, lungs, kidney, and brain. We also have periodic acceleration therapy, which like all of our equipment generates growth factors that encourage new tissue growth, which is used for repair and restoration of diseased and/or damaged organs and tissues.

DR. KONDROT: I'd like you to talk about some of the misconceptions about stem cell therapy. Some people feel that it should be illegal. What is the current status? Who can do it? Let's talk a little bit about that.

DR. STEENBLOCK: I think the most important thing to clarify is that when we're treating patients with stem cells, we're not using aborted fetal tissues or embryonic tissues. We are using the patients' own stem cells from their bone marrow. In other countries, we have associations with physicians who are using stem cells obtained from the umbilical cord of newly born, healthy babies. The cords are rescued before the umbilical cord is thrown away. The stem cells from these fresh human tissues are then analyzed for diseases and if no toxicity is found, they are processed for treatment. These physicians have used umbilical cord stem cells, umbilical cord wall stem cells, and stem cells from the placenta and from the amnion, which is a membrane of the amniotic sac.

There are also stem cells from a patient's fat tissue. Fat stem cells are obtained by first doing a mini-liposuction where small amounts of fat are removed from abdominal wall fat.

Those stem cells are very good if prepared correctly. So many doctors are claiming to be doing fat stem cells, but they don't have a stem cell lab and are using a "kit" which is supposed to be able to help the doctor make proper stem cells. In my experience, these kits often don't work well, and the doctor lacks the skill to determine if the cells they are preparing are done correctly or not. It is much better to find a physician that has his/her own lab and trained doctor-level lab technicians to do the actual stem cell separation from the fat in an absolutely sterile manner. These fat stem cells are called mesenchymal stem cells, which suppress the inflammatory processes in the body and take away pain and misery. For autoimmune disease, arthritis, and repairing joints, they work very well. These mesenchymal stem cells are also in bone marrow. Mesenchymal cells taken from bone marrow, fat, or umbilical cord all work well.

In addition, stem cells can be used for neurological disorders. For example, in cerebral palsy, bone marrow stem cells are absolutely fantastic for repairing the brain. See the following videos for some great success stories with the use of stem cells for cerebral palsy.

- www.youtube.com/ watch?v=I40yUlcdNwQ

- www.youtube.com/ watch?v=zyGsmTfKMZc

- www.youtube.com/ watch?v=OY9Jgbzlz5k

- www.youtube.com/ watch?v=sweldtmVeBo

DR. KONDROT: I have a basic question for you. What makes a stem cell special? Why can it be so beneficial in helping treat a lot of these conditions that you mentioned?

DR. STEENBLOCK: That's a very good

question. Basically, it's hard to describe the chemistry, biochemistry, and physiology of a stem cell. What we can say is that it is the most primitive cell in the body. It is used by the body to make any and every kind of tissue. A real stem cell can form muscle, nerve, bone, connective tissue, epithelial tissues, and new cells for the intestinal tract, brain, kidney, heart, spleen, liver, and lungs. It has this tremendous potential of being able to create new cells and tissues.

How does it do that? It does that on the basis of instructions by the tissue in which it is placed. If we inject stem cells into a damaged kidney, in general, that damaged kidney will tell the stem cells what kinds of tissues the kidney needs to rebuild the organ. The stem cells will then rush into the kidney's damaged tissues and start to generate new nephrons, glomeruli, blood vessels, or whatever that tissue needs for its repair. That goes for all the other organs, whenever they are injured or diseased.

Stem cells have this primitive ability. They're like this clean slate and can be utilized by the body for fixing virtually any kind of tissue that has damage or disease present. Our job is to make sure that the person gets enough of the right kind and numbers of stem cells to the problem areas. Highly potent stem cells are cells that are most able to invade into the damaged tissues, take up residency, grow, proliferate, and make new tissues. We want cells that are fresh, have long telomeres, can successfully engraft, can

make new tissues vigorously, and can generate a lot of growth factors because a lot of our patients are older. Older patients do not have many, if any, growth factors.

If you look at the number of growth factors in a baby's umbilical cord, there are about 10,000 micrograms per deciliter of growth factors. In a 90-year-old there are about 100 micrograms, and 10,000 versus 100 is why a young baby can double in size during the first month of life and the old person cannot repair even minor cuts and injuries much less the damage from a stroke or heart attack.

The number of growth factors in an older person is negligible. To get good repair and regeneration in these patients, we need to give them a large number of very vigorous stem cells that have a lot of growth factors because the stem cells need these growth factors. We have to give the older person a lot more stem cells than we do a younger person.

2. If we give healthy, fresh stem cells to a person with cerebral palsy, the patient and family will most likely see improvements.

For example, in my stem cell therapy book, I have a number of cases of cerebral palsy (CP). Generally, CP is like a mini-stroke or a brain injury at birth from a lack of oxygen. This can cause paralysis and often great muscle spasticity where the person cannot walk or function well. If we give healthy, fresh stem cells to a person with cerebral palsy, between a few hours to two to three weeks, the patient and family will most likely see improvements. The spasticity starts to decrease by up to 80%, which is so much improvement that the child can then walk and use his/her arm(s) again. It is really great to see children be able to feed themselves for the first time ever. Stem cells are often the miracle these patients and their families have been longing for. I've even seen those who are blind regain their eyesight. Some of the patients start to walk again. Why is that? It's because we have given them so many growth factors and stem cells that their damaged tissues are able to grow and repair themselves very well.

DR. KONDROT: Dr. Steenblock, as an expert, you're the one who can evaluate the disease and determine which stem cells are best for the treatment and then also support it with various growth factors. It's not as simple as it seems. It's not a magic bullet for everyone. It does take some evaluation and treatment, especially in people who are older and have complicated intractable diseases. Let's talk a little bit about what cases, morphology, and diseases seem to respond the best to stem cell therapy.

DR. STEENBLOCK: I've had great results with cerebral palsy. We have had good results with autism with bone marrow treatments and really good results with multiple sclerosis with umbilical cord stem cells in other countries. With ALS, amyotrophic lateral sclerosis, we

have very good results, but each case is different. I have discovered the underlying causes of the spontaneous forms of ALS and know how to treat it effectively, but if the person waits too long it is always difficult or impossible to reverse long-term damage to the spinal cord. If anyone is interested in stem cell treatments for amyotrophic lateral sclerosis, I have videos on YouTube:

- www.youtube.com/
  watch?v=4dH6DldYzCw

- www.youtube.com/
  watch?v=f12xLlqPBeE

- www.youtube.com/
  watch?v=bXSKyI9W-
  po&feature=c4-overview&list=UUd
  SWCyftv7tlGovEXODnFXw)

These videos describe what I believe is its etiology. I also have a PowerPoint presentation that we would be happy to send to people. It describes my understanding of the causes and how to treat this terrible condition. My colleagues generally do not agree with me when they first hear about my discoveries, but, if they follow my program, they can achieve remarkable results, using my teachings.

With joint and arthritic problems where there are damaged joints, fat stem cells and bone marrow stem cells are very good, and umbilical cord stem cells are excellent. With the neurological cases, stem cells are good for conditions like stroke and traumatic brain injury. I recently treated an elderly gentleman who had suffered from a stroke. He had made great progress with previous stem cell treatments, but his right hand continued to be spastic and frozen in a fist. I administered stem cells into his back and within one hour, he had regained the use of his right hand. His results are now posted on youtube.com as well. (www.youtube.com/watch?v=bXSKyI9W-po&feature=c4-overview&list=UUdSWCyft-v7tlGovEXODnFXw).

In those cases with the older person, we often administer the stem cells into the cerebrospinal fluid or intranasally. With the intranasal procedure, the stem cells are given through the nose so they go directly into the brain. That method is good for Parkinson's, Alzheimer's, and frontal lobe dementia. Usually I try to use both methods in order to maximize the entry of the stem cells into the brain. In older people with these diseases, we have to use a lot of cells and the younger and fresher, the better.

Autoimmune diseases are due to infectious diseases but often include yeast infections and heavy metal poisoning from mercury, iron, cadmium, lead, etc. With a lot of autoimmune diseases like rheumatoid arthritis, the infections need to be cleaned up, and any metal toxins need to be removed. Any of these (infections, metals, toxins) all irritate the immune system and propagate the autoimmune problem. The cleaner the body, the less disease one has!

We try to clean out the body as much as possible and then give stem cells. With this procedure of cleansing the system and then giving the stem cells, there is a good chance of the patient going into remission. There are a lot of different tricks that we use that can help the patients improve.

DR. KONDROT: I want to talk a little bit about the use of stem cells for stroke victims. I observed first-hand a personal friend of mine, a young individual, who had a massive stroke. His recovery after the use of stem cells was just remarkable. I couldn't believe the success. Talk a little bit about your approach because not only do you use stem cells but you use hyperbaric oxygen, too.

DR. STEENBLOCK: I pioneered the use of hyperbaric oxygen for strokes in a total rehab program that included hyperbaric oxygen treatments (HBOT) daily for 60 days. The HBOT sessions last an hour and a half and are taken five days a week, which is a lot of treatment and a lot of time. The patients had to come to Mission Viejo and live here for two months. That's a lot of time out of a person's life.

With stem cells, now the patients can come for one week, two weeks, or three weeks. If they stay for three weeks, they have time for hyperbaric oxygen treatments that increase their growth factors and stem cells, and we see better overall results. In general, the more treatments that increase the activity and number of stem cells and growth factors in the person's damaged brain tissues and the longer these treatments are given (minimum of three weeks), the better the results. It takes three weeks for new blood vessels to grow into the damaged brain and that is essential for the repair of the damaged brain.

Now, of course, the younger you are, the better your stem cells are as well. You get better results if you're young. If you're really old, then unfortunately, you need to consider that the golden years require you to spend more gold. Older people with a number of problems require lots of fresh, healthy stem cells and growth factors because that's what it takes for an older person to have good recovery. If you are older and your only problem is the stroke, then often only one treatment is needed to get good results, but the treatment must be an injection directly into the cerebrospinal fluid.

3. The best results with stem cells are achieved when they are given within the first ten days after a stroke.

For that matter, this is the best time to give cells for any type of acute injury like a heart attack, etc. If only one injection can be given, then the optimum time is 72 hours after an acute injury like a stroke, but they can be given anytime after the stroke. The longest time after a brain injury that I treated successfully with stem cells was 50 years! This 63-year-old male was partially paralyzed and had difficulty speaking since a car accident at the

age of 13. I gave him stem cells into his spine, and he experienced good improvements in both his speech and walking within one month after the treatments. We were all amazed since I had told him that it almost certainly would not help at such a late date after his injury.

When it's given soon enough, there is the chance of very good results but even then, the more stem cells that are given, the better the results. It can mean the difference between greater wellness and being paraplegic, being in a wheelchair, not being able to talk or function, and not having quality of life after a stroke. I have some patients who have the stem cell treatments and are able to walk and talk again, but if they had not done the treatments, they more than likely would have died or had been permanently disabled with a terrible lifestyle. Quality of life is really what is important and stem cells are really great at improving that quality.

Some patients with acute strokes who have had substantial amounts of stem cells given to them may still have a limp or speech impairment, but that's a far cry from not being able to speak and just sitting in a wheelchair or living in a bed. Of course, there are cases where the damage is so severe and so massive that nothing can help but when the patient and family think there is a chance for recovery, the use of stem cells should be strongly considered.

It's a very effective therapy. We've treated hundreds if not thousands of stroke patients with stem cells. There are also strokes that affect the eye. We haven't talked about that, but that's another situation that is treatable if we can treat them right away. In people with cortical blindness, which other doctors have given up on, I have had success. The problem with this condition is that the treatment needs to be long enough. Usually I would recommend the two-month course of hyperbaric oxygen along with stem cells, brain growth factors, external counter-pulsation, autohemotherapy, etc.; then my success rate on these "incurables" is about 70-80%.

It's really important that when you are dealing with these serious conditions like stroke to get on the telephone and call me right away, so we can give you the best advice on treatments.

Another type of problem, generally for older people, is macular degeneration. I think the reason why most people get macular generation is because they are not getting enough oxygen to the back of their eyes especially at night.

My way of treating macular degeneration is the exact opposite to conventional medicine. The macula is the part of the eye that you use to focus. The center of this macula is the exact point, which is used by your eye as you read this. This is the "fovea" and this tissue is the most metabolically active tissue in your body. As such, it requires more oxygen than any other part of your body. With aging, your blood vessels get tortuous, hardened, and corroded. These changes occur to the blood vessels that supply oxygen to the respiratory centers in the base of your brain. These changes slowly cause damage to these breathing centers, and this process results in sleep apnea and intermittent bouts of lack of oxygen at night, which is when your heart rate and metabolism slow down. Now when the macula and fovea experience a lack of adequate levels of oxygen, their cells do what all living cells do when they are being deprived of oxygen: they start to secrete new blood vessel growth factors to help grow new blood vessels so they can get more oxygen.

This is great if these growth factor signals are continuous day and night since, within three weeks, you would have new blood vessels to the macula, and the macula would not degenerate. Unfortunately, the growth factors are produced only intermittently since the oxygen deprivation comes and goes depending on your activity, your diet, and the way you sleep at night. If you have any kind of infection in the sinuses, this can interfere with the oxygen and growth factor signals as well. All of these spell trouble for the new blood vessels the macula is trying to generate, so that more oxygen can be delivered. This intermittent stimulation creates intermittent growth of the cap-illaries which results in imperfect blood vessels. These tiny capillaries begin to form but then die back when there are not enough growth factors. This creates weak and leaky blood vessels, and this then is what causes the macula to degen-erate, i.e., the combination of lack of oxygen and imperfect leaky blood vessels.

Now the standard eye doctor knows that the leaky blood vessels are the problem so he/she gives you a shot of Avastin or Lucentis ($4,000) monthly to stop these capillaries from continuing to try to repair the macula. *But* what if you give the macula good healthy continuous new capillary growth factors 24 hours per day? What happens is that the eye is able to repair itself and heal itself. Your vision improves and the problem goes away!

The problem with this natural way of treating is that eye doctors are not used to looking for and treating the cause of macular degeneration. They don't want to look into these alternative types of treatments since they can make good money doing what all of the other eye doctors do. Medicare even pays for these expensive treatments, but won't pay anything for actually fixing your damaged blood vessels to make you healthier! What we alternative physicians do is give growth factors and stem cells on a daily basis in a consistent manner. That allows the tissue of the fovea and the macula to make new blood vessels on a daily basis in a normal fashion.

After a few weeks, new blood vessels will form that are healthy. The results are new healthy blood vessels in the eye and improvement in vision. In many cases, this treatment even cures the macular degeneration. Then the macular degeneration is stable for years after that. I use hyperbaric oxygen, stem cells, external counterpulsation, and chelation. All of these treatments have been shown to work again and again with most of my patients.

There are failures, of course, but often these failures are due to problems the person has that have not been addressed. For example, of 36 consecutive macular degeneration patients, I did CT examinations of their sinuses and 50% of these definitely had a chronic sinus infection with absolutely no symptoms. These infections stop stem cells from entering into and fixing the macula, so sinus problems need to be identified and treated first if we are going to be able to fix the macular degeneration! Not correcting nighttime lack of oxygen is another chronic problem that needs to be consistently treated, usually by supplemental oxygen.

DR. KONDROT: The key points that Dr. Steenblock has gone over is that people tend to do better if it's an acute problem, when they seek stem cell treatment soon after the episode. Also, it depends on your age. The younger you are, the better the results will likely be. Your book, *Umbilical Cord Stem Cell Therapy*, is an easy read. It really helps explain the differences among all the different types of stem cells. You have some great case examples in that book. I highly recommend it. Let's talk about the product that you've researched and developed called Stemgevity, which is a very interesting product. Can you explain what the product does?

DR. STEENBLOCK: It has a lot of different ingredients, including seaweed. The seaweed is a special kind of sulfated mucopolysaccharide. It has the ability to release stem cells. We went through all the different products we could find and tested all of them. We put the ones that are the most effective for stem cell mobilizing into this product. Stemgevity has other properties besides stem cell mobilization and proliferation. It actually helps to produce better stem cells and allows them to be released from the bone marrow into the blood circulation. We see in one week about a 300% increase in the number of stem cells circulating in a person's blood. One of the kinds of stem cells that are released is a very small embryonic-like stem cell, which is the most primitive stem cell we have in our body. It's present in the bone marrow and tissues.

It's very small, less than 1 micron in diameter, which is one-fifth the size of a red blood cell. When you have damaged tissue and capillaries, the capillaries are squeezed together because of the damage and swelling. These tiny cells are able to penetrate through these damaged blood vessels into the damaged tissue. We can get regeneration in damaged tissue with the very small embryonic-like stem cells (VSEL cells) where, otherwise, normal stem cells cannot get in because of the lack of blood flow. That's a very important aspect of regeneration: getting the stem cells into the area that needs repair. These VSEL cells are a new and exciting concept in medicine.

Our Stemgevity is very powerful. It allows those small stem cells to be released to fix the damaged tissues. We see that with stroke patients. They actually see improvement in their paralyzed arm or leg. They actually see improvement with the use of this product. In addition to its action with stem cells, Stemgevity has anti-bacterial and anti-viral activity. This product is good for treating and preventing the common cold. So it is a helpful adjunct to other cold treatments you may be taking.

It also has some anti-coagulant activity. If you have an older person who has a lot of atherosclerosis (hardening of the arteries) and poor circulation, Stemgevity is a very good product for helping with these conditions. It also helps prevent blood clots in the legs. You can take from 1 capsule up to 15 capsules a day. You can change the dose depending on how it makes you feel.

Sometimes, you can feel pretty tired from the Stemgevity because it stimulates your growth factors. When we were children and had a lot of growth factors, we also needed more sleep. This is one of the side effects you see with Stemgevity and with stem cells. When stem cells are given to a patient, they may need to sleep more because the body is producing more growth factors. The need for more sleep also occurs with Stemgevity because more growth factors are being produced. That means it is working. Just try to get extra sleep when you're tired. Don't force yourself to keep on going. If the fatigue is really bad, just cut back on the number of capsules and it will reduce the production of growth factors, and the fatigue will go away. If you do experience tiredness, that's a good thing because it means that you are growing and repairing tissue. That's part and parcel of the regenerative process. Whenever I give stem cells and the patient is having a lot of fatigue a week or two weeks later, I always tell them that is a good sign. It really is because it means they're going to see good improvement.

DR. KONDROT: Is this product only available by a doctor's prescription?

DR. STEENBLOCK: It's over-the-counter. You can order it through www.Stemgevity.com, or you can call our office and order it from our office at 1-800-300-1063. The cost varies. If you take one pill a day, the cost is less than $30 a month. If you take more, then of course, it will cost more. If you have serious conditions, you should take more such as 3 to 12 per day. If you're trying to recover from an acute trauma or a car accident where there is tissue to repair, you may want to take more capsules. If you're an alcoholic and want to get off of alcohol, you can take two, three, or four capsules a day because that will help you stop drinking. It also helps with hangovers. It's amazing what it does because it has so many benefits. It has a little bit of lithium, so it has anti-depressant activities because lithium also stimulates the release of stem cells. It also has a lot of these other properties.

DR. KONDROT: I personally use it in my practice. It's a great product. The only caution I have is that there's no substitute for good medical advice. Dr. Steenblock is one of the top doctors focusing his practice on stem cells. He is definitely the expert.

....

DAVID A. STEENBLOCK, DO AND
ALEXANDER THERMOS, DC, DO
Personalized Regenerative Medicine
26381 Crown Valley Parkway, Suite #130
Mission Viejo, CA 92691
(800)300-1063
(949)367-8870
www.stemcellMD.org
www.stemgevity.com

Jerald Tennant, MD, MD(H), PSc.D

IRVING, TEXAS

Interviewed November 10, 2013

1. **You can do surgery or take medicine, but you will not get rid of your chronically painful dysfunctional area if you can't make new cells.**

2. **Humans are portable electronic devices.**

3. **Voltage measurements become abnormal long before blood tests become abnormal, and blood tests tend to become abnormal before you have symptoms.**

DR. KONDROT: Dr. Jerry Tennant, started out as an ophthalmic surgeon, just as I did. We have another thing in common. We were both early investigators for the Excimer laser. Dr. Tennant was investigating the VISX laser, and I was investigating the Summit laser. Of course, that goes back quite a few years. Let's begin with your story. How did you make that transition? I remember when I was beginning to use intraocular lenses and doing surgery, you were a man who was well respected in the ophthalmic community.

You had developed your own intraocular lens. I think you were the first one to have an outpatient surgical center. You were on literally the cutting edge. Tell me about the transition you had from ophthalmology to being a leading doctor in integrative and alternative medicine.

DR. TENNANT: I did a lot of the research for the laser called VISX when we were beginning to do what most people now think of as Lasik. I had a lot of fun doing that, but what I didn't realize at the time was that the laser would not kill viruses.

One patient in particular was a fellow who had corneal scarring. He also happened to have leukemia. I was using the laser to remove the superficial scars from his cornea. As those cells were removed and exploded, the viruses were released but not killed. They apparently came up through my mask and nose and into my brain, so I developed encephalitis.

The symptoms that followed affected me so that I could see a patient and know what was wrong with them, but I couldn't remember how to write a prescription. I also developed spastic movements, which doesn't really work well if you're operating inside somebody's eyeball. I also developed a bleeding disorder and my platelet count dropped down to dangerous levels where I was bleeding under the skin. For all those reasons, I had to quit work at the end of November 1995. I went to the best physicians I could find in the country. They basically said, "You have three viruses. We don't know what to do about it, so don't call us. We'll call you."

I was at home and sleeping about 16 hours a day. I had about two or three hours a day in which I could think clearly enough to understand a newspaper. Then it was like a light switch would go off, and I couldn't understand it anymore. During those two or three hours a day in which I could think, I realized I had to try to figure out how to get myself well because I couldn't find anybody else who could help me. That's how I began.

DR. KONDROT: That was really a big shift. Your story is similar to mine. I came down with severe adult-onset asthma. It almost killed me a couple of times. Traditional medicine didn't help me. When I discovered homeopathy, one homeopathic remedy cured my asthma and got me off all my medicine. Maybe you could share with us what in particular convinced you that there was much more to understanding disease than what traditional medicine teaches us.

DR. TENNANT: During those two or three lucid hours a day that I had, I developed the idea that if I could figure out how to make one cell work, I could make them all work. Even though I hadn't done so for 30 years, I bought a bunch of books on cellular biology and started reading them. One of the things that jumped at out me from each of them was there would either be a paragraph or page in the books that said cells have to run at a pH of 7.35 to 7.45. I didn't remember very much about pH, so I started reading about it again and discovered that pH, other than being about acid-base balance, was really just a measurement of voltage in a solution.

If you think about a copper wire that's going to my computer, the telephone, or whatever, if the switch is on, electrons are flowing. If the switch is off, electrons stop flowing. In a solution, you have a totally different situation in which the solution can be an electron donor or electron stealer. What you do is you use a sophisticated voltmeter and measure the voltage of the solution. That voltmeter will tell you if it's an electron donor or electron stealer. Then you convert the measurement you get to a logarithmic scale between 1 and 14. That's called pH.

By convention, minus 400 millivolts is considered a pH of 14. Minus is meant to be an electron donor. Plus 400 millivolts of electron stealer is the same thing as a pH of zero. If it's neither a donor nor a stealer, then it's called a pH of 7. When we say that cells are designed to run in an environment of 7.35, that is a synonym of minus 20 millivolts of electron donor, and 7.45 is a synonym of minus 25 millivolts of electron donor.

Obviously, it jumped out at me that cells need to have energy to work. That seemed obvious. By the way, people get confused about this voltage thing because any cellular biology book will tell you that cells have to run in an environment of minus 20 to minus 25 millivolts. If you put an electrode inside the cell and outside the cell and measure across the cell membrane, you'll get as high as minus 90 millivolts. When you read that cells are running at minus 90 millivolts, they're really talking about cell potential from inside to outside the cell, but the environment has to be minus 20 to minus 25.

That really was the beginning of being able to figure out how to get well. Of course, the next question to confront me was, "How do I measure it?" I eventually discovered that a chap named Nakatani was the first person to use modern electronics to measure acupunc-ture meridians. He published his work in 1951.

I got his rather rudimentary equipment and began to measure. I discovered that my brain was running between 2 and 4 millivolts. Thus, I knew why it didn't work. The next question was, "What am I going to do about it?"

I eventually discovered some Russian technology that was available that had a particular wave form that would transfer electrons to cell membranes. That was called the Scenar device. I acquired one of those and began working on myself. Pretty soon, my brain started working again. That was the turning point for me being able to get myself going again and begin moving down the path of understanding how the body really works instead of the way I was taught.

DR. KONDROT: Your cells did not have enough electrical potential to function. No matter what the traditional doctors did, they just couldn't get the engine to turn over because you didn't have any battery.

DR. TENNANT: That's right. A new Mercedes is not going anywhere without a battery, is it?

DR. KONDROT: Your book is called *Healing is Voltage: The Handbook*. It's a wonderful book. For those of you who are interested in this aspect of regaining your health, I would highly encourage you to buy his book. Dr. Tennant, you were talking about voltage and the necessary potential for cells and our bodies to exist. I wonder if you could discuss how much energy we need just to maintain our body functions and how much energy we need if we're going to be regenerating our body and making new cells.

DR. TENNANT: As I mentioned before, cells require minus 25 millivolts to run, but in order to make a new cell you need to have minus 50 millivolts. If you think for a moment about my thumb or your thumb, assuming it's a good thumb, it's running at minus 25 millivolts.

Now you hit it with a hammer. You've destroyed some of the cells. The thumb will automatically go to minus 50 millivolts once it realizes there has been damage. One of the things that happens at minus 50 millivolts is that it dilates arterial capillaries. The reason we're designed that way is those capillaries need to dilate so they can dump the raw materials at the curb, so to speak, so you can start building new cells to repair those you damaged with the hammer.

When those arterial capillaries dilate, you notice several things. One is you have a throbbing thumb. Secondly, you have swelling. Third, your thumb is red and warm and it makes you say bad words. You have all the ingredients, minus 50 millivolts and all the raw materials, and you get busy making new cells. Pretty soon you've replaced all of those you smashed with the hammer. Now your thumb goes back to being nice and pink

and functional again. The pain is gone and you have a perfectly good thumb again. That's the way we're designed.

1. You can do surgery or take medicine, but you will not get rid of your chronically painful dysfunctional area if you can't make new cells.

However, if you hit your thumb and you don't have enough voltage stored in your body to get up to minus 50 millivolts, or if you can get up there but you run out of voltage before you finish making new cells, your thumb will drop to some other voltage less than 50 millivolts, and now you're stuck in chronic disease. Let's say your thumb is at 15 millivolts. You can do all the surgery you want or take all the medicine you want, but you will not be successful in getting rid of your chronically painful dysfunctional thumb because you can't make new cells. What that teaches us is that chronic disease occurs when you lose the ability to make new cells that work.

DR. KONDROT: The question I have is what are those contributing factors that prevent the body from making the necessary voltage?

DR. TENNANT: One of the things that people don't appreciate is how often we have to make new cells. Cells simply wear out very frequently. You get new cones in the macula of your eye every two to three days. The lining of your gut is replaced every three days. The skin you're sitting in tonight is only six weeks old and your liver is eight weeks old. We're constantly wearing our cells out and making new ones. In addition, if you have injuries like hitting your thumb with a hammer, or if you have infections or toxins that damage cells, you have to make new ones.

If you can make new cells that work, then you stay well, but when you lose the ability to make new cells that work, then you have chronic disease. Chronic disease can only be reversed when you have all of the things necessary to make new cells.

That leads us to the question: what does it take to make a new cell that works? First of all, I mentioned that you need to have 50 millivolts of voltage. The primary things that cause low voltage are inadequate amounts of thyroid hormone because thyroid hormone controls the voltage of every cell membrane and every mitochondrion. Next, we have dental infections because the teeth are wired into the circuits that we'll describe in just a moment. If you have a dental infection, that shuts down the voltage. A scar across the power circuit will create a short or a ground and toxins.

The thing you have to do to identify why you can't make new cells is to start with measuring the voltage so you know what the voltage is and how inadequate it is. Of course, you can do that with things like my biomodulator. The Tennant Bio-modulator is a little handheld device that is about the size of a computer mouse. It allows you to tap onto certain points, basically the battery poles of the energy supply to whatever organs are functioning, and measure its voltage.

You need to have the voltage. You need to have the raw materials that it takes to make new cells. The insides of cells are made from amino acids, except for the neurons or the nervous system. Fifty percent of the inside of the nervous cells is cholesterol. The primary source of amino acids to make new cells is stomach acid because the human is designed to never ever absorb whole proteins. You must only absorb amino acids, and that occurs when you eat a protein, and stomach acid breaks it into amino acids. Critical to staying healthy is to have adequate balance of stomach acid so that you have on ongoing source of amino acids to make the inside of cells.

The outside of cells are made of special fats called phospholipids. In order for you to have those available, you need to have a functional liver and gallbladder because it takes bile, which is manufactured by the liver and stored in the gallbladder, to have the fats available to make the outside of cells.

Next, you need to have vitamins and minerals. It turns out that the ability for vitamins and minerals to enter the cell is controlled by a substance called fulvic. Then, you need to have oxygen, which turns out to be controlled in the body by a substance called nitric oxide.

Of course, you need to have water because cells are 70% water. The water that is inside the cells is in a special form. It's not just H20; it's actually H302, which is specialized water. Just drinking other substances doesn't easily give you that substance. Then, of course, you have to deal with the toxins.

DR. KONDROT: I'm particularly interested in the idea of scars interfering with voltage, so I hope you can address this. We've had many other guests on the show talk about the thyroid, dental amalgams, and toxins, but let's talk about how scars on your body can interfere with electrical conduction in the body and how they can contribute to our body's inability to heal. This is something interesting and new to me.

2. Humans are portable electronic devices.

DR. TENNANT: To understand scars, we have to set the stage for how the body is wired. One of the things that people have to begin to conceptualize is that as humans, we are portable electronic devices. If you think about any portable electronic device, it needs to have a portable battery pack in order for it to work. Since we are not tethered to something, we need to have an ongoing source of energy of electrons to keep all of the things in our bodies working.

It turns out that our portable battery packs are our muscles. First of all, you have to understand the word piezoelectricity. If you stress certain substances, they emit electrons. For example, if you take a piece of quartz and squeeze it with a pair of pliers, it emits electrons and that

phenomenon is called piezoelectricity. It turns out that our muscles are piezoelectric, so every time you move your muscles, they generate electrons. In addition, the neat part of this system is that they are also rechargeable batteries. Whenever you move around, you begin the process of not only generating electrons but also recharging your portable battery pack, namely your muscles.

It turns out that every organ in the body has its own stack of muscle batteries, so the muscles are all surrounded by a fibrous sheath called a fascia. Fascia are what are known in electronics as semiconductors. What we have then is a stack of rechargeable batteries much like you would have inside of a flashlight, but surrounding those batteries is a semiconductor that will move the electrons from those batteries only in one direction. A semiconductor is an assembly of atoms in such a way that there are excess electrons that can move easily and quickly from one to the next but only in one direction.

Because our fascia are semiconductors, we now can understand why, if you put a drop of essential oil on your big toe, in a nanosecond the frequency of it is already up at your brain because the movement of electrons through semiconductors is amazingly rapid.

The way we're wired is that our muscles or battery packs then begin in either a hand or a foot. For example, the so-called spleen acupuncture meridian actually begins down in the big toe and then it goes to the soleus muscle and the lower leg. At the knee, it attaches to the sartorius muscle, which goes up to the hip where it attaches to the external oblique muscle. That attaches to the pectoralis minor muscle. Then that connects to its corresponding battery pack, which is called a stomach acupuncture circuit.

That begins up around the eye, so there is the orbicularis oculi, which goes around the eye and then it goes down the masseter muscle and down the sternocleidomastoid to the sternalis muscle to the rectus abdominis. It keeps going down into the leg through the rectus femoris and the quadriceps. Then you are down to the tibialis anterior and then into the foot.

Now you have one battery pack that goes from the foot up and the other one comes from the head back down. That is the battery pack that supplies all of the organs that are wired to it. Not only does it get spleen and stomach, but it also gets most of the things going on in the exterior portion of the eye. It gets the front lobes of the brain, etc.

When you have someone with chronic disease, the first thing you want to do is ask the question, "What is the battery pack for that organ?"

For example, if you're having heart disease, you want to know what the battery pack for the heart is. Once you learn what they are, the flexor carpi ulnaris and the biceps brachia, the teres minor and the subscapularis, etc., then you can measure that battery pack and see why the voltage is so low that you can't make

new cells to keep your heart fixed.

DR. KONDROT: The muscle strength and the muscle mass are directly related to the energy of the battery pack. Is that what you're saying?

DR. TENNANT: Absolutely. People who don't exercise don't recharge their batteries. If you don't recharge your battery pack, that organ has to try to get by on an inadequate amount of voltage not only to do its day-to-day function, but it runs out of adequate voltage to make new cells. Therefore, you end up with chronic disease.

Once you begin to think like an electrician instead of a physician, you begin to figure out how and why people are sick. One of the problems is that each of these battery packs and its fascial wiring runs through a tooth. Unfortunately, an infected tooth functions just like the circuit breaker does in your home. When you have an infected tooth and it shorts out, then it shorts out that battery pack. Therefore, that thing doesn't work.

I've already shared with you my personal history of how I got sick. The reason that I didn't have enough voltage in my system for my brain to work is because I had a root canal in tooth #14, which is the upper left molar. That was a circuit breaker that shut down my spleen/stomach circuit, so instead of having 25 millivolts in the frontal lobes of my brain, I now had between two and four millivolts. That's why it didn't work and why it kept getting worse. It was because I couldn't make new cells.

In my particular case, the primary reason that I got sick was a root canal tooth. I also, as it turns out, had hypothyroidism, which contributed to that. It also turns out that I had a scar. Here's how all of that fits together. Our teeth have a pump inside of each tooth that pumps fluid from inside the tooth into the mouth. This was proven by dental researchers at Loma Linda in California where they would inject dye into various parts of the body, and within six minutes the dye was in the pulp of the corresponding tooth. Within 30 minutes it was in the mouth.

These pumps require a reasonable amount of voltage to work, and when you put a scar across an acupuncture circuit, or in other words when you put a scar across the fascia of that tooth's power supply, that pump malfunctions. When that pump malfunctions, you get decay in that tooth.

Decay is more a function of lowering of the voltage in the power supply of the circuit than it is how many sweets you eat and how many times you brush your teeth. What happens then is that the pump quits working and you get a filling. A few years go by, and you get another filling. A few more years go by, and you get a crown, and then you get decay under that crown which goes unrecognized or the tooth begins to hurt enough that the dentist does a root canal.

Now, you have enough infection in that tooth that it flips that circuit breaker, which takes the power down adequately to cause the organ that's attached to that battery pack to malfunction because it can't keep itself healed, and it doesn't have enough voltage to run day to day.

If you do the timeline, you will see that often people fell off their bike when they were six years old and got a scar, which caused a tooth to decay. Eventually, 30, 40, or 50 years later, they have a tooth that acts like a circuit breaker and now the voltage drops and they have organ failure. When the voltage drops to plus 30 millivolts, you get cancer.

DR. KONDROT: How do you treat the scars?

DR. TENNANT: You can easily fix the scars by using an essential oil blend that I've put together that has the appropriate essential oils to treat scars. You put a little of the oil on there, and then there's an attachment that creates a specific magnetic field that goes into the biomodulator. In two to three minutes, you will fix the scar. You can prove that it's now working by measuring the voltage or by muscle testing it. Now, you know that the scar has been fixed, and it is permanent about 98% of the time.

DR. KONDROT: Could you tell us a little bit about the device that you developed called the biomodulator. Listeners know that I'm a big advocate of microcurrent, pulse electromagnetic field, and all of the devices that put electrons back into the body. Your device is very unique, and it's a little bit different from microcurrent or the pulse electromagnetic field.

DR. TENNANT: The device I developed and use is called the biomodulator and it has an attachment called a biotransducer. I mentioned earlier that when I was trying to get well, I discovered a Russian device called a Scenar, and that's what I began to use. As I began to understand how things worked more and more, I began to believe that I had figured out some frequency sets that might be more beneficial than the Russian one.

A couple of things happened. One of them is that I discovered that the Russian frequency set wasn't unique to the Russians. We actually found devices from the state of Maryland from the late 1800s that had the same waveform in it, so this waveform was not unique to Russian development.

Secondly, I did figure out ways to modify that basic pattern into frequency sets that I thought would be more effective and more efficient. As it turns out, that's basically true. Many people who have both devices, and/or other devices, find that the biomodulator seems to be more efficient at getting the job done as far as transferring the electricity or the electrons that are necessary to make things work.

In my device, I have some very specific frequency sets. One is designed for musculoskeletal problems, and one is designed for organ systems, and it's automated.

My professional device also has frequency sets that operate when you detect that various regions of the body are not in electronic resonance as they should be. Within just a few minutes, you can put them back into resonance. Then the body can communicate with itself appropriately. It's sort of like having a television set with lots of incorrect imagery on it. You go in and tune it and make it in resonance, and now you have a perfect picture. We can now do that to the body with the more advanced device and its more advanced frequency sets.

Basically, the way I work is when I see somebody who has a chronic illness, the first thing I want to do is what's called turning on the cranial sacral pump, which you can do with specific points on the side of the neck. Then, you want to check to see if the valves between the esophagus and stomach, the stomach and the small intestine, and the small intestine and large intestine are stuck open, as they often are. Using the biotransducer you can quickly close those so they're functional again.

Then, you measure a specific point on the body that tells you what the voltage is in each of the organs. Knowing which organs have normal voltage or which ones are actually running at 50 millivolts, which means they're trying to heal something, or which ones are low, which means they can't heal, allows you to know which battery packs are not working.

Next, you begin the process, as any electrician would, of figuring out why the voltage is low. You're most commonly going to find some combination of hypothyroidism, dental infections, and scars. Then you start fixing those things. One of the things about the biomodulator is that not only does it have the ability to measure and tell you what has low voltage, but it also has the ability to switch into the therapeutic mode where you can actually begin to insert electrons and recharge the battery packs so that those organs can begin to function again.

DR. KONDROT: The machine is both a diagnostic and a therapeutic piece of equipment. It helps you diagnose the problem, whether you're electron deficient or there are excessive electrons, and then you can correct it.

3. Voltage measurements become abnormal long before blood tests become abnormal, and blood tests tend to become abnormal before you have symptoms.

DR. TENNANT: By simply measuring your personal voltages in your power packs every day, you can quickly pick up when something is going amiss and begin to fix it before you have symptoms or organ failures.

I know this may be new information to many readers, but there's a lot of informa-tion on my website. My website is www.TennantInstitute.com. You can also get my book, *Healing is Voltage,* on Amazon or from my website. I have another book called *Healing is Voltage: Healing Eye Diseases,* which discusses how to use electronics in eye problems.

DR. KONDROT: You also are an avid lecturer. Maybe you could tell us a little bit about the courses that you offer around the country.

DR. TENNANT: I begin on a Thursday evening at 7:00 and give a basic overview of things. It's sort of like we've discussed here, but of course a bit longer and in more detail. Those are open to the public. On Friday and Saturday, I teach not only how to use the biomodulator but how to get well by measuring voltage in stomach acid and all of these other things. Details about the course are at www.SENERGY.us

....

JERALD TENNANT, MD, MD(H), PSC.D
9901 E. Valley Ranch Pkwy, Suite 1015, Irving, TX 75063,
(972)580-1156
jtenn@tennantinstitute.com
www.tennantinstitute.com

Books by the
Top 20 Alternative Doctors

Most are available through Amazon; also check the author's website to order.

GABRIEL COUSENS, MD, MD(H)
The Rainbow Green Live-Food Cuisine
There Is a Cure for Diabetes, Revised Edition: The 21-Day+ Holistic Recovery Program
Depression-Free for Life: A Physician's All-Natural, 5-Step Plan
Conscious Eating
Spiritual Nutrition: Six Foundations for Spiritual Life and the Awakening of Kundalini
Torah as a Guide to Enlightenment
Creating Peace by Being Peace: The Essene Sevenfold Path
Tachyon Energy: A New Paradigm in Holistic Healing
www.drcousens.com

LEE COWDEN, MD, MD(H)
Alternative Medicine Definitive Guide to Cancer
Co-author of *Cancer Diagnosis:*
    What to Do Next
Detoxify Your Home and Body
Foods that Fit a Unique You
Longevity: An Alternative Medicine Definitive Guide
www.acimconnect.com

EDWARD KONDROT, MD, MD(H), CCH, DHT
10 Essentials to Save Your Sight
Healing the Eye the Natural Way
Miracle Eye Cure? Microcurrent Stimulation
www.HealingTheEye.com

JAMES LEMIRE, MD
The Ultimate Guide to Natural Health, the Premier Handbook for Natural Health in the 21st Century
www.LemireClinic.com

KARL ROBINSON, MD
Small Doses Big Results: How Homeopathic Medicine Offers Hope in Chronic Disease
www.homeopathyyes.com

ROBERT ROWEN, MD, MD(H)
Defeat Cancer: 15 Doctors of Integrative & Naturopathic Medicine Tell You How
Second Opinion's Complete Healing Library (Volume One)
9 Alternative Health SCAMS
www.doctorrowen.com

FRANK SHALLENBERGER, MD, MD(H), ABAAM
Bursting With Energy: The Breakthrough Method to Renew Youthful Energy and Restore Health
The Type-2 Diabetes Breakthrough: A Revolutionary Approach to Treating Type-2 Diabetes
www.antiagingmedicine.com

MARK STARR, MD, MD(H)
Hypothyroidism Type 2: The Epidemic
Hypothyroidism Type 2: The Epidemic Updated 2011 added: Hashimoto's & Graves' edition
How to Prevent Heart Attacks
www.21centurymed.com

DAVID STEENBLOCK, DO
Umbilical Cord Stem Cell Therapy: The Gift of Healing from Healthy Newborns
www.stemcellmd.org

JERALD TENNANT, MD, MD(H), PSCD
Healing is Voltage: The Handbook
Healing is Voltage: Healing Eye Diseases
www.tennantinstitute.com

Index